BIPOLAR BATTLE PLAN

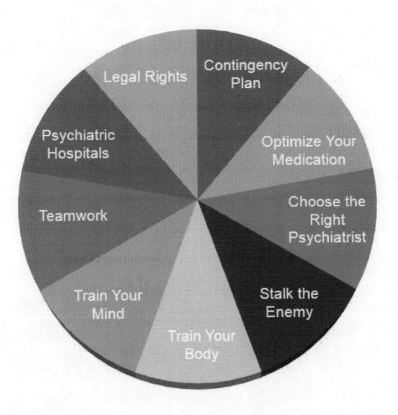

BIPOLAR BATTLE PLAN
Fighting the War against Bipolar Disorder

TROY GILLEM

iUniverse LLC
Bloomington

Bipolar Battle Plan
Fighting the War against Bipolar Disorder

Copyright © 2013 by Troy Gillem.

All rights reserved. No part of this book may be used or reproduced by any means, graphic, electronic, or mechanical, including photocopying, recording, taping or by any information storage retrieval system without the written permission of the publisher except in the case of brief quotations embodied in critical articles and reviews.

The information, ideas, and suggestions in this book are not intended as a substitute for professional advice. Before following any suggestions contained in this book, you should consult your personal physician or mental health professional. Neither the author nor the publisher shall be liable or responsible for any loss or damage allegedly arising as a consequence of your use or application of any information or suggestions in this book.

iUniverse books may be ordered through booksellers or by contacting:

iUniverse LLC
1663 Liberty Drive
Bloomington, IN 47403
www.iuniverse.com
1-800-Authors (1-800-288-4677)

Because of the dynamic nature of the Internet, any web addresses or links contained in this book may have changed since publication and may no longer be valid. The views expressed in this work are solely those of the author and do not necessarily reflect the views of the publisher, and the publisher hereby disclaims any responsibility for them.

Any people depicted in stock imagery provided by Thinkstock are models, and such images are being used for illustrative purposes only.
Certain stock imagery © Thinkstock.

ISBN: 978-1-4759-9867-2 (sc)
ISBN: 978-1-4759-9868-9 (hc)
ISBN: 978-1-4759-9869-6 (e)

Library of Congress Control Number: 2013916697

Printed in the United States of America

iUniverse rev. date: 09/27/2013

CONTENTS

Acknowledgments xi
Introduction xiii

Chapter 1 What's at Stake? 1
                Startling Bipolar Statistics 1
                Episode from Hell: The Hospital Roof 4
                Trained and Untrained 8

Chapter 2 The Good News 11
                Positive Personality Traits Common to
                    Bipolar Individuals 11
                Recognizing Our Rare Abilities 14

Chapter 3 Contingency Plan 17
                Creating Your Contingency Plan 17
                The Role of Your Psychiatrist 20
                When to Launch Your Contingency Plan 20

Chapter 4 Optimize Your Medication 25
                Accept That You Need to Take Medicine 26
                Bipolar, Heal Thyself 27
                Dial In Your Medications 30
                Beware of Side Effects! 35
                Medicine Noncompliance 39

Chapter 5 Choose the Right Psychiatrist 41
                Rating a Psychiatrist 43

      Psychotherapy (Talk Therapy) 44
      Finding a New Psychiatrist 45
      No-Cost Initial Appointments 46
      Getting the Most Out of Appointments.............48
      When to Get a New Psychiatrist.......................51

Chapter 6 Stalk the Enemy 53
      What Is Bipolar Disorder?..................................54
      Bipolar Episode Triggers...................................59
      Bipolar Disorder Is Predictable 63
      Bipolar Disorder Facts and Statistics................65
      Causes of Bipolar Disorder...............................67

Chapter 7 Train Your Body..73
      Exercise Several Days a Week 73
      Get Fresh Air..74
      Stretch Several Times a Day 74
      Build the Core 74
      Use Alcohol and Drugs Intelligently 75
      Make Love 75
      Take Vitamins 76
      Drink Water...76
      Eat Healthily...76
      Get Your Thyroid Checked...............................77
      Natural Herbs and Spices.................................77
      Take Showers or Baths.....................................78
      Brush Your Teeth and Use Mouthwash............78
      Shed Extra Pounds..78
      Animal Lovers 79

Chapter 8 Train Your Mind 81
      The Path with Heart...82
      Death Is Stalking You..83
      Always Do Your Best 84

    Self-Importance Is Your Greatest Enemy 86
    Stalk Yourself 89
    Erase Personal History 91
    Autosuggestion 92
    Face Fear Head On 94
    Running the Bipolar Marathon 96

Chapter 9   Teamwork 99
    Again, You Aren't Alone 99
    How Can the People Closest to You
        Help You Manage Your Illness? 101
    Arm Your Team with Your Contingency Plan 107

Chapter 10 Psychiatric Hospitals 109
    Advice from Fellow Bipolars 110
    Reasons to Check into a Psychiatric Hospital 112
    Voluntary Check-in 113
    Involuntary Commitment 113
    How Hospitalization Can Help 114
    What You Need to Know about Psychiatric
        Hospitals 115

Chapter 11 Legal Rights 117
    The Laws Governing Involuntary
        Commitment 117
    Legal Rights When in the Psychiatric
        Hospital 121
    Can I Be Forced to Take Medication? 123
    How Do I Get Discharged from the
        Hospital? 123
    The Benefits of Having a
        Psychiatric Advance Directive 124
    The Americans with Disabilities Act 126

Chapter 12 Winning the Bipolar War **127**
　　　　　Bipolar Battle Plan Summary 128

Helpful Resources **129**
Bibliography **133**
Appendix **137**
My Personal Contingency Plan **141**
Personal Notes **145**

This book is dedicated to the men and women throughout the ages who, despite being bipolar, carved their way to greatness.

Also to my kids, Jennifer, Rachel, Jeremy, and Natalie who are a constant source of inspiration.

ACKNOWLEDGMENTS

First and foremost, I must thank the many bipolar individuals who graciously agreed to be interviewed on an anonymous basis about their experiences and struggles with bipolar disorder. Their advice, stories and anecdotes are included throughout the pages of this book, illuminating the reality of being bipolar.

I would also like to express my gratitude to the many people who saw me through the writing of this book, provided support, talked things over, read, wrote, offered comments, allowed me to quote their remarks, and assisted in the editing, proofreading, and design.

INTRODUCTION

I wrote this book with the intent of helping those who are suffering from bipolar disorder. Helping doesn't necessarily mean coddling, however. You must take personal responsibility for managing your illness. Bipolar disorder is a condition that can't be ignored or underestimated. The implications are simply too serious: suicide or living a crippled, limited life, handicapped, with personal and professional relationships undermined.

The first step is accepting that you aren't alone. Take a look at this list of many notable individuals who have survived and thrived with symptoms of this disorder. Note that they are listed in alphabetical order because bipolar disorder doesn't discriminate based on gender or race, income or upbringing: Ludwig Van Beethoven, Russell Brand, Jim Carrey, Drew Carey, Dick Cavett, Winston Churchill, Kurt Cobain, DMX, Salvador Dali, Jean-Claude Van Damme, John Denver, Patty Duke, Charles Dickens, Richard Dreyfuss, Carrie Fisher, Larry Flynt, Harrison Ford, Vincent van Gogh, Ernest Hemingway, Kay Jamison, Billy Joel, Meriwether Lewis, Abraham Lincoln, Kristy McNichol, Marilyn Monroe, Isaac Newton, Florence Nightingale, Jane Pauley, Edgar Allan Poe, Theodore Roosevelt, Sting,

Troy Gillem

Ted Turner, Brooke Shields, Ben Stiller, Mark Twain, Mike Wallace, Robin Williams, Owen Wilson, and Virginia Woolf.

Remember that these are only some people who are brave enough to admit that they are bipolar or known to cope with symptoms of bipolar disorder. Millions suffer daily. Struggling alone, oftentimes afraid to confess to others or confront their condition, too many go unnoticed and untreated until it's too late.

Myself included. I am bipolar, having struggled more than twenty years and all too aware of what it takes to confront and "cure" this disorder. I have survived three major episodes, which resulted in three visits to a psychiatric hospital, one due to a suicide attempt. All the while, I have maintained a career in engineering, obtained a master's degree, and currently work as a technical writer for an aerospace company. I am also the proud parent of four awesome kids. This goes far beyond me, though.

The idea of creating a bipolar battle plan began while witnessing my dad's struggles with bipolar disorder, his manic highs, and his much more devastating depressions during which he would sit in front of the television for months at a time, existing only to eat and sleep. He never sought help or stayed on medicine to battle the illness. This was a travesty. No one deserves this kind of life, and I am passionate in my belief that it should not happen to you or anyone else.

As you will read, I have had to confront my darkest thoughts and demons in order to write this book. It wasn't easy. Seven years ago, I attempted suicide. Today I have found balance and achieved security by creating this "battle plan." I have successfully used the plan over time to remain episode free and advance toward achieving my dreams.

Know that this book was written to help. So please note that neither the publisher nor I can be held responsible or liable for any loss or damage allegedly arising as a consequence of your use or application of any information or suggestions contained in this book. The information, ideas, and suggestions in this book are not intended as substitutes for professional medical advice. You should not undertake any diet or exercise regimen or follow any recommendations in this book before consulting your personal physician.

Everyone is different, but this disorder and how it affects us is consistent. We experience ups and downs sometimes so severe that feeling utterly average would be welcome. Good days—waking without that uninvited guest lurking, waiting to pounce—at times seem so rare. It is a struggle to be productive, to gain the trust and respect of others, but most of all, to trust that things will get better, that this episode will pass, yet there will be another battle in the future. There are no quick fixes. Accept that this is a lifelong struggle requiring immediate attention and long-term remedies.

Armed with a battle plan for bipolar disorder, you and those who care about you will be ready for the worst and, more important, at last embrace all that life has to offer.

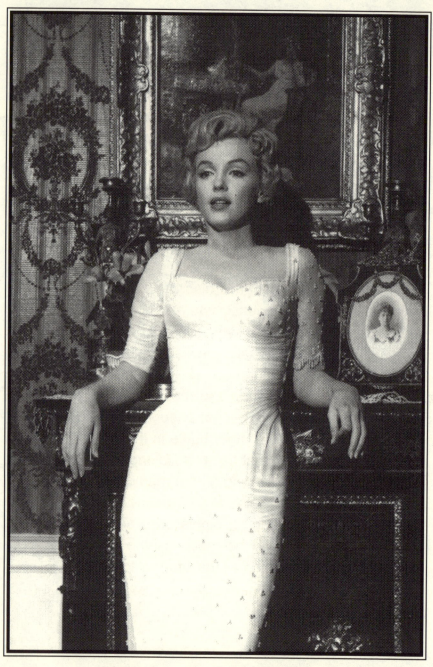

I wish I knew why I am so anguished.
—Marilyn Monroe, actress, 1926-1962

CHAPTER 1
What's at Stake?

Dyin' ain't much of a livin', boy.
—Josey Wales, *The Outlaw Josey Wales*

Startling Bipolar Statistics

Your life is at stake. And you are your own worst threat. Studies show that approximately 30 percent of people with bipolar disorder (manic depression) attempt suicide. It is unbelievable that one out of three of us try to kill ourselves! One out of five of these suicide attempts are successful (fatal). This is the highest suicide rate of any psychiatric disorder (Novick and Swartz 2010).

Besides suicide, other catastrophic outcomes of bipolar episodes include the following:

- physical violence
- self-mutilation
- financial disaster
- loss of job and damage to a person's career
- loss of spouse or romantic partner

- alienation of children
- loss of friendships
- loss of self-respect

In addition, bipolar illness is associated with severe health issues:

- The life expectancy of an adult with bipolar disorder is approximately fifteen years shorter than that of a person without it (Cowen 2011).
- Approximately 25 percent of bipolar individuals are obese (McElroy 2002).
- Forty percent of people with bipolar disorder struggle with alcohol and drug abuse (Evans 2000).
- Bipolar individuals are three times more likely to be diabetic than the general population (Thompson 2010).

In her book *Madness: A Bipolar Life*, Marya Hornbacher captures the essence of bipolar disorder.

> Here's the hell of it: madness doesn't announce itself. There isn't time to prepare for its coming . . . . It shows up without calling and sits in your kitchen. You ask how long it plans to stay; it shrugs its shoulders, gets up, and starts digging through the fridge . . . . In the early years, it's like a switch flips on, and though only a moment before you were totally sane, suddenly you have gone mad. But as you learn to manage madness, you begin to notice sooner that it's on its way. (Hornbacher 2009, 225)

How do we battle a disease that has the ability to take control of our thoughts and emotions and cause our minds to deceive and betray us? How do we overcome an illness that has the power to cause us to attempt suicide, start banging our heads against the wall, and spend money recklessly, not to mention so many other destructive acts? How do we surmount the health issues caused by bipolar disorder, such as a much shorter life span, obesity, diabetes, and abuse of drugs and alcohol?

The best solution is to follow a lifelong battle plan like the one shown in figure 1. This bipolar battle plan consists of nine "weapons," each of which can be deployed as necessary to fight the war against the enemy, better known as bipolar illness.

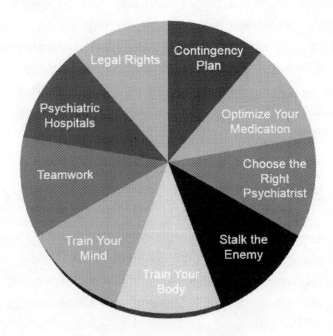

Figure 1: Bipolar Battle Plan

Winning invariably involves contingency plans, and yours will be *the most important weapon* you will have against your bipolar illness and uncontrollable episodes. No athlete or army goes unbeaten; this book offers personal experiences and tried-and-true steps to confront this condition.

Therefore, in order to better prepare you for the pitfalls and the ups and downs that are the only things guaranteed in life, the end of this book offers a "Personal Contingency Plan" for you and those close to you to create and share. Make several copies and give them to your "team"—primary and secondary contacts (psychiatrist, family and good friends)—so they know how to respond when it is essential.

The final pages of this book are for personal notes on ideas and emotions that may pop into your head while reading. Feel free to fill these pages with any questions or concerns that arise, and they will become invaluable to revisit over time. Not only will you have a tangible way of tracking how your battle plan has evolved and changed you and your life, but you will also have a priceless document that captures all you were upon finding this book when you finally started taking steps to find your true self.

Episode from Hell: The Hospital Roof

I was surrounded. Eight security guards were securing my arms behind my back with handcuffs. The leader, the one in charge, was breathing fast and was extremely pissed off. "Bend him over the table and pull down his pants," he instructed the others.

I went berserk, biting a huge piece of flesh from someone's forearm, butting my head against a guard's face, and fighting with all the strength I had. The guards subdued me, bent me over a steel table like you would see in a morgue, and pulled down my pants. I began sawing my wrists forcefully on the steel of the handcuffs, back and forth, back and forth, as hard and as fast as I could. I wanted to die. Getting raped was not an option. I felt the most excruciating pain imaginable in my wrists as they became slick with blood—unending, unrelenting, the worst hell I ever imagined.

I woke up in a hospital bed feeling like my arms had been cut off. They were purplish, and I remember thinking I had new arms attached, and I saw an IV attached to the left one. It was then that I remembered what happened. I squeezed my anus to see if it was sore, but it wasn't. Thank you, I thought. I then carefully checked out the rest of me: wiggled my toes, flexed my knees, and lifted my head off the pillow. I felt for my penis with my right hand, and then I felt something coming out of its tip. My heart accelerated to top speed and adrenaline began to flow like lava from an erupting volcano. Lifting the covers I saw a plastic tube entering the urethra. My enraged eyes followed the tube to see where it went, finding a bag filled with yellow fluid I recognized as urine.

"What is going on?" I screamed.

A pretty black nurse came through the door of my room. She noticed that I was looking under the covers and said, "It's a catheter tube. How are you feeling?" She checked the IV that was connected to my left arm, writing on her clipboard as she examined me and chatting away, adding, "You sure did give us a scare." She told me the doctor would be here soon to talk to me.

My mind scrambled to remember how I had gotten to the hospital. Such a blur . . . Then it hit me like a sledgehammer. I had swallowed all of the pills in my bottles of Lithium and

Seroquel. The next thing I could remember was being wheeled on a stretcher into the emergency room of the hospital. I lay on the stretcher for a little while, and then a nurse walked toward me with a needle in her hand. When I saw her face, I recognized her. The irony—she had slept overnight on my couch a few nights earlier. I had met her and her girlfriend at a bar and asked them to come back to the pool at my apartment complex and swim. I had had great sex with her hot friend in my bedroom while this "nurse" with the needle slept on my couch. I had no clue at the time, remembering only her saying that she worked in a women's prison. But there she was, masquerading as a nurse getting ready to plunge a needle into me. I freaked out, jumped off the cart, ran around the corner, and crouched down with my back against the wall. A security guard yelled, "Hey!" and started running toward me. The image of him running around the desk and coming toward me was the last conscious memory I had prior to waking up in the hospital room. I must have resisted. One guy could not have subdued me, not in that state.

The nurse came back into the room and removed the catheter tube—quick pain, then relief and a sense of freedom. Once more, the nurse said the doctor would be in to talk to me soon. Then she smiled at me and left. Everything seemed out of sorts. I tried to get it straight in my head. I had attempted suicide, been transported to the hospital in an ambulance, freaked out when I recognized the nurse in the ER as the prison guard who had slept on my couch a few nights earlier, sawed my wrists off so I wouldn't get raped by eight guys, and woke up in a hospital room with a catheter tube in my johnson and an IV in my arm. Where was the freaking doctor?

I looked at the open window. It was about six feet high and didn't have a screen. I decided to vamoose. So I yanked the IV needle out of my arm. All I was wearing was hospital pants, with no shirt or shoes. I got up out of bed and went to the window. I used the crank handle to open it as much as I could and then grabbed the window with both hands and pulled hard. There was a loud creaking of metal on metal, something broke loose, and the window opened wide enough for me to slip through.

At that moment, a couple of nurses came running through the door of my room yelling, "What are you doing?"

I slipped out of the window and stepped down about two feet onto the flat roof of the hospital. It was rock-and-roll time, and I ran like the wind. After about twenty or thirty strides, however, I was out of roof. Looking down and seeing a seven-foot drop to the roof below, I decided there was no stopping me now. I jumped, landed barefoot, dropped and rolled, and kept running. I then ran out of roof again, and it was about a twelve-foot drop to the ground this time. I got myself down by turning my body backward and easing myself down so that I was holding onto the edge of the roof with my hands and then dropping to the ground below. Onward I went, tearing ass across the parking lot toward the adjacent neighborhood.

I was free!

This is my own story. Shocked yet? Note that I initially didn't want to reveal that I had gotten so low, attempted suicide, and had to be involuntarily hospitalized. Accepting that I had a problem was the first step. I was picked up later that day by the police and taken to a psychiatric hospital, where I was involuntarily committed.

The cause of this episode was that I had decided that I was tired of feeling like a "robot" and had stopped taking Lithium. Several days later, I started having bipolar symptoms. I started sleeping a lot less, had racing thoughts, and quit eating. Things escalated quickly after that. I began having psychotic thoughts and lost control of my mind. As a result of this catastrophic episode, I promised myself that I would not quit taking medicine again without making a plan with my psychiatrist. Also, together with my psychiatrist, I created a contingency plan that has saved me twice in the past three years.

Trained and Untrained

There is no such thing as tough; there's trained and there's untrained.

—Creasy, *Man on Fire*

Warcraft of all types must be mastered. Developing expertise and proficiency in fighting against bipolar disorder is probably the most important trade for you at points in your life. I am giving you a call to arms to become a bipolar warrior. Fight and claw and scratch with all of your strength, courage, and willpower to overcome the bipolar beast that invades your mind and wants to destroy you. This is the most difficult and important undertaking you will ever face.

Precious moments have already been snatched from your life by the enemy, and it will only try to steal more—if you allow it to. Make the decision to win the war against bipolar disorder no matter what. Winning means you will decrease and eventually eliminate your bipolar episodes as well as making your dreams come true.

The book you are holding in your hands promises one thing: to provide you the weapons and training to fight bipolar illness strategically, intelligently, and as a warrior. By making a true effort to master the weapons in your bipolar battle plan, you will be well armed to achieve victory. This is your life—you don't get another!

If you remember only one thing from this book, remember this: do not give up. Don't you ever give up! ☺

CHAPTER 2

The Good News

Positive Personality Traits Common to Bipolar Individuals

Okay, enough bad news! Let's get to the good stuff.

Take heart in the fact that when bipolar episodes are not occurring, individuals with bipolar disorder are busy living their lives, often excelling at their professions, being moms or dads and students, just like anyone else. In fact, many bipolar individuals currently living or who have lived in the past will be remembered as successful individuals who left legacies of greatness and fame.

Despite a deep depression throughout his life, Abraham Lincoln saved the United States and freed millions from chains. Winston Churchill summoned the strength to inspire a world at war, never bowing to the Nazis or depression. Beethoven gave us the most moving music ever to grace ears; Van Gogh and Dali blessed our eyes with surreal paintings, so bright and expressive; Ernest Hemingway captured a lost generation in words; Edgar Allan Poe perhaps channeled his demons to give us tales of horror.

Florence Nightingale pioneered battlefield nursing, while Marilyn Monroe reinvented the notion of beauty. The people who make us laugh out loud are oftentimes bipolar, including Ben Stiller, Drew Carey, and Robin Williams. Look around—bipolar people are striving daily; despite their condition, they are bringing the best out of themselves. They have carved their paths through life, and so can you.

A study published in the *Journal of Affective Disorders* in February 2011 found that having bipolar disorder may enhance specific psychological characteristics that are generally viewed as valuable and morally or socially beneficial. The authors reviewed eighty-one studies that noted positive characteristics and identified five qualities associated with bipolar patients: creativity, realism, spirituality, empathy, and resilience. The conclusion was that encouraging an appreciation of the positive aspects of bipolar disorder could help combat the stigma and improve patient outcomes (Ghaemi 2011).

Common Personality Traits

Creativity: The link between bipolar disorder and creativity is well established. Visual arts, performance, writing, and music—bipolar talent in all the arts is common and sometimes exceptional.

Exuberance: Exuberance is an abounding, ebullient, effervescent emotion. It's a celebration of the passion and joy in mania and hypomania. It's contagious, starting with that person who makes everyone smile.

Hypersexuality: Lust is also a prominent feature of mania. People with bipolar disorder tend to be dazzling, passionate, and adventurous lovers.

Emotional Perspective: What goes up must come down—and then go back up again. Viewing life and issues from both ends makes bipolar individuals more philosophical about the meaning of things. It also gives perspective they didn't have before.

Depth of Experience: You'll not meet more experienced, well-traveled, multidimensional people. They have exceptional and often unusual stories to share. People with bipolar disorder, who are so often adventurous, tend to be high-achievers and leaders with above-average intelligence.

Depression: What's good about depression? you most surely will ask. Light needs shadow, and the most profound understanding includes both. People with bipolar are complex and can illuminate the whole human experience.

Resilience: After suffering through tragic bipolar episodes, bipolar individuals' act of resurrecting themselves gives them the resilience to handle most anything else that comes their way. Bring it on!

Courage: Tied in with bravado and grandiosity, at its most severe, courage can entail dangerous risk-taking. Yet at its best, courage is rare, inspiring, and heroic.

Recognizing Our Rare Abilities

We have created masterpieces, won wars, and led countries. Is this condition really holding us back? Some have succumbed to the challenge—Kurt Cobain comes to mind immediately—while the vast majority of us have achieved a "new normal" to lead the lives we have always wanted. What's unique to bipolar individuals is the reality that our condition, once controlled, can give us enhanced abilities, strength, and an unrelenting attitude to achieve far more.

A broken bone heals much stronger than before; a soldier's mettle is tested in battle, making him or her come out more capable. Once aware of our condition and its challenges, we can then be aware of the early signs and confront. No longer naïve, we are ready for all of life's challenges—and its myriad opportunities.

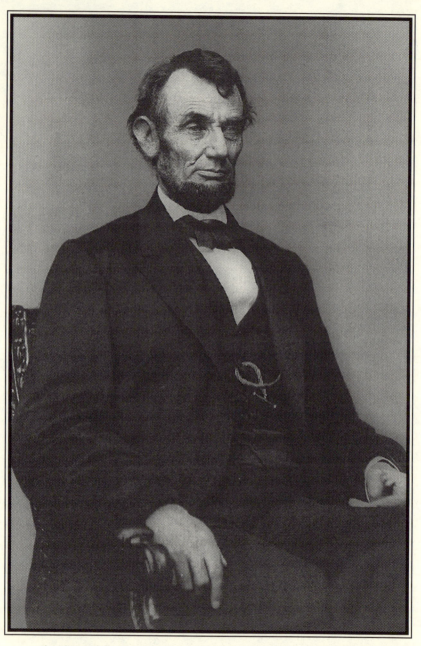

In the end, it's not the years in your life that count. It's the life in your years.

—Abraham Lincoln, president

CHAPTER 3
Contingency Plan

A wise man has taught me to always have a contingency plan.

—Abraham Lincoln

The purpose of the contingency plan is, first, to safeguard you from having a bipolar episode and, second, to help you avoid catastrophe if you do have one. When it becomes hard to ignore your manic or depressive symptoms, that's the moment you must do something about them. Bipolar episodes escalate like wildfire, so a rapid response is everything. The stakes are too high to allow yourself to slide into a bipolar episode of disastrous proportions.

Creating Your Contingency Plan

This chapter outlines how to create a contingency plan, the role your psychiatrist plays in it, and when to put your contingency plan into action. My story in chapter 1, "The Hospital Roof," drives home how important it is to have a contingency plan in place and ready to execute. Equally important is creating a team that is aware of your contingency plan, should you need their help when it is critical.

"Jane" (name changed to protect identity and to allow her to speak openly) tells how she created her contingency plan.

I asked my psychiatrist whether I could call her at 2:00 a.m. if I were experiencing bipolar symptoms. She said, "Yes, absolutely, anytime twenty-four/seven. If I am not available then another doctor in my practice will be on call." We discussed what steps to take if I started to have an episode. She told me one thing I could do immediately was adjust my medication. I am currently taking 400 milligrams of Lamictal in the mornings and 600 milligrams of Lithium and 200 milligrams of Seroquel at bedtime. She told me if I start to have noticeable bipolar symptoms to increase my Seroquel dosage to 400 milligrams for several days. She also told me to carry Seroquel with me and if symptoms became severe to take some immediately, even if I have to chew it.

Jane then offers how she shared her contingency plan with others to ensure it would be put to use.

Another thing I did was asked two people I trust implicitly to be part of my contingency plan. I asked my sister, an ex-alcoholic, whom I am very close with. She knows how to deal with mental adversity and has been sober for five years. I also asked my best friend, Liz. They are both aware of my disease and told me to call day or night if I need help. The final thing I did was put my contingency plan in writing.

Jane's Contingency Plan

When I begin having bipolar symptoms I will take the following actions:

1) Adjust my medication dosage(s) per the prearranged plan I made with my psychiatrist.
2) Call my psychiatrist and make an appointment to see her ASAP or talk to her on the phone.
3) Call the person (people) I have recruited to be part of my contingency plan.
4) Distance myself from my loved ones if I feel agitated, violent, or out of control so they are safe.
5) Check myself into the hospital if things get bad enough.
6) Carry extra medicine with me and take it immediately if symptoms start getting out of hand.
7) Remove myself from stressful situations.
8) Ensure I am getting sufficient sleep. If not, I will call my doctor and request a sleep aid.
9) Start taking my medications if I am not currently taking them.
10) Stop drinking alcohol and/or taking illegal drugs or at least slow down the pace.
11) Exercise and get fresh air every day.
12) Take vitamins and eat healthy.

Create your own personal contingency plan and put it in writing using the form at the end of the book. Give copies to your team—primary and secondary contacts (psychiatrist, family, and good friends) and talk to them about what they should do if you launch your contingency plan.

The Role of Your Psychiatrist

The most important function of your psychiatrist is to be there in your time of crisis, which is why he or she gets paid the big bucks. You must be able to count on your psychiatrist to help you immediately, day or night, if you contact him or her for help. This means talking to you on the phone or seeing you in person. If he or she is not reachable, then another on-call doctor must be available twenty-four/seven. If you think you need help, don't hesitate to call your psychiatrist!

When to Launch Your Contingency Plan

Monitoring yourself for out-of-the-ordinary moods, thoughts, and feelings is a must, not an option, to managing your bipolar illness. If you notice symptoms that persist for several days, it is a warning siren that you had better get a handle on what is going on—pronto! If things seem to be getting worse, not better, launch your contingency plan before the episode gains steam. It is imperative that you take immediate action by increasing your medication, making an appointment with your psychiatrist, or both.

Gary (again, name changed) tells about using his contingency plan to keep from going off the deep end.

> I began going manic in September when the leaves were changing. Fall is historically when my episodes rear their ugly head. My episodes ramp up slowly and unnoticeably, and I start getting really happy, busy, horny, and emotionally intense at the same time.

I really love these periods in my life, and it's hard to believe anything out of the ordinary is happening. Then suddenly, I reach the point where I become psychotic. This one time, I was convinced I was being followed by some Mexicans who were part of a drug cartel and wanted to kill me. I began taking evasive tactics like making sure I wasn't being followed so they wouldn't discover where I lived. I got to the point where I was scared to go to sleep and stayed awake all night holding a shotgun. One morning, I was lucid enough to recognize I needed help and called my friend Chris, who previously had agreed to be part of my contingency plan. He realized I needed help and convinced me to call my psychiatrist. My doctor prescribed a stronger medicine, and I was able to calm down and fortunately rid myself of psychotic thoughts in a few days without having to go to the hospital.

A list of early warning signs for both mania and depression follows. These may indicate the onset of a manic or depressive bipolar episode. If you are having troublesome symptoms, it is time to execute your contingency plan.

Mania Early Warning Signs

- similar pattern of symptoms from previous episodes
- heightened mood, exaggerated optimism and self-confidence
- sleep disturbance
- grandiose delusions, inflated sense of self-importance
- increased physical and mental activity and energy
- excessive irritability and aggressive behavior
- racing speech and thought, irrational ideas

- impulsiveness, poor judgment, and distractibility
- delusions and hallucinations, such as a direct connection to God
- increased sex drive
- compulsion to keep talking, unusually sociable
- jumping from thought to thought or project to project
- aggressive or fast driving
- impulsive purchases
- reckless behavior, such as spending sprees, sexual indiscretions, or alcohol and drug abuse
- increased interest in risk-taking activities like gambling
- feeling bulletproof or endowed with special powers or qualities
- impatient or frustrated by the slowness of others
- paranoia or hallucinations
- argumentative, picking fights

Depression Early Warning Signs

- similar pattern of symptoms from previous episodes
- sleep disturbance
- suicidal thoughts
- avoiding or withdrawing from others
- abandoning activities you usually like
- not answering your phone or replying to e-mails
- continually having negative thoughts
- prolonged sadness or unexplained crying spells
- loss of energy
- changes in appetite
- paying less attention to personal appearance, hygiene, and grooming
- social withdrawal/isolation
- increased feelings of worry and anxiety
- feelings of guilt or hopelessness

- little interest in sex
- inability to concentrate or make decisions
- unexplained aches or pains
- slowed and more difficult thinking
- paranoia or hallucinations
- self-loathing

Your body and mind are giving you clues that "All isn't well—prepare!" Once these early warning signs are understood and identified, mania and depression are far more easily handled. Those "downs" won't be so severe, and so getting back "up" won't take so long. The mania and depression can be managed. The battle is underway, and you're already on the winning side.

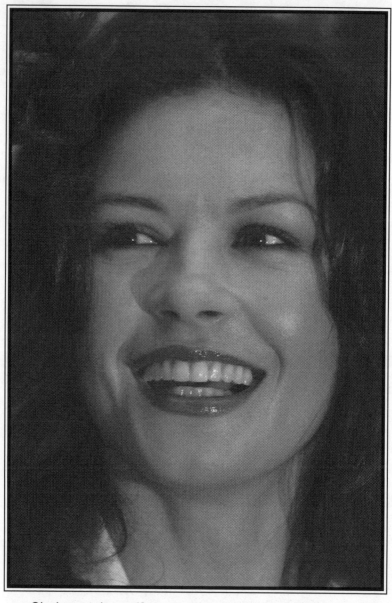

She's got herself worked out with her meds and she's raring to go!

—Michael Douglas (husband)

—Catherine Zeta-Jones, actress

CHAPTER 4
Optimize Your Medication

Up there, we gotta push it. That's our job.
—Viper, *Top Gun*

This chapter details how to determine the best medications and corresponding dosages to effectively battle your bipolar illness and achieve optimal mental and physical health.

Like heart disease or diabetes, bipolar disorder is a biological illness, and, most often, medication is required to treat it. Medication can bring your mania and depression under control and prevent relapses once your mood has stabilized. Bipolar disorder has a number of different symptoms, reflecting difficulties in several different areas or systems of the brain. Different medicines target different brain functions. You may need medicines to help stabilize your mood, curb manic symptoms, relieve depressive symptoms, manage anxiety, control psychosis, improve information processing, and compensate for side effects.

It takes skill, finesse, and guts galore to determine the specific medications that effectively combat your bipolar disorder. Just as it takes time and practice to learn golf or a new language, learning how to use the powerful pharmaceutical pills on the market to your advantage is a skill that improves with experience. It is your job to push the limits of your medications in order to find the "sweet spot" where you are mentally sharp and focused; have plenty of get up and go, a positive attitude, and no bipolar symptoms; and are happy with yourself and your life.

This isn't easy. It would be awesome if the first time you are prescribed medicine to treat your bipolar illness, the medicine worked great, suppressed your symptoms, and kept you from having future bipolar episodes. However, this is rarely the case, and it is more likely that adjustments will need to be made to your medications as time goes on. Don't be afraid to take calculated risks in making changes. You do not want medications to make you feel mediocre; you want them to make you feel great!

Accept That You Need to Take Medicine

People with bipolar disorder are reluctant to admit there is a problem. It takes most of us more than one bipolar episode before we are convinced that we actually have a problem. The more pain, agony, and disruption to our lives that is caused by a bipolar episode, the sooner we become "believers." It is a landmark event when you accept that you are bipolar and need to take medication on a daily basis to treat your illness. When you accept that medicine is necessary to minimize symptoms and avoid future episodes, you can turn the energy you have been expending rejecting the medicine and channel it into finding the medications that work best.

You must be your own judge and jury to determine whether you need to take medicine on a daily basis—no one else is in a fitting position to do so. Make the decision based on the ramifications of having another bipolar episode and also on optimizing your health, happiness, and life.

Bipolar, Heal Thyself

You are the general of your own individual bipolar battle plan. Your psychiatrist will prescribe you medications, but you are the only one who can tell if they are working. You must become an expert at treating your own disease. Live by the motto, "Bipolar, heal thyself."

Strive to find the best combination of medicines to treat your disease just as heart patients or cancer patients search for the right medicines to treat their diseases. Learn to monitor yourself closely and keep an eye out for bipolar symptoms. Collaborate with your psychiatrist regarding the medications. Learn how to rate your medications and tweak the dosages based on how you feel mentally and physically.

While medication is the foundation of bipolar disorder treatment, therapy and self-help strategies also play important roles. You can help control your bipolar symptoms by exercising regularly, getting enough sleep, eating right, monitoring your moods, keeping stress to a minimum, and surrounding yourself with supportive people. Living with bipolar disorder is challenging. But with medication, healthy coping skills, and a solid support system, you can live fully while managing your symptoms.

Jane relates some of the actions she takes to avoid bipolar episodes and manage her well-being.

> To help me avoid bipolar episodes, I exercise, eat fairly healthy, and take vitamins. I make sure to go out of my house and talk to someone at least once a day, even if it is just at a Starbucks. I also have once a month appointments with my psychiatrist, spend time with my kids and friends, and most importantly, not drink alcohol more than once or twice a week.

Become Your Own "Mental Detector"

Many diseases can be detected by some kind of medical test—for example, blood tests for diabetes and kidney function and CT scans for brain tumors—but there is no test that can detect bipolar disorder. The telltale signs are bipolar symptoms, major mood changes, and bipolar episodes.

The onset of a bipolar episode is not readily apparent to anyone other than you. Episodes start slowly, oftentimes unnoticeably, and they pick up speed as the days go on. You must be astute enough to recognize that you are experiencing bipolar symptoms and strong enough to take appropriate action. Because no one else knows your thoughts, feelings, and inherent behavior patterns like you do, it is crucial that you become your own "mental detector." Monitor your thoughts, moods, and energy levels on a regular basis.

Ask yourself the following questions:

- Have I laughed today?
- Do I feel like myself?

- Am I looking forward to something coming up in the future?
- Did I barely drag through the day?
- Am I having any psychotic thoughts?
- Am I depressed?
- Am I manic?

As soon as you notice bipolar symptoms, take action ASAP! Allow no delays—there is no time to lose! This may mean increasing your medication and making an appointment with your psychiatrist. If things are bad enough, launch your contingency plan.

Substitute Medicine for Alcohol and Drugs

An important statistic to keep in mind is that approximately 40 percent of bipolar individuals abuse alcohol or drugs. For many of us, it is an attempt to self-medicate. Instead of seeking health care, we use drugs or alcohol to mask uncomfortable feelings. There's a cultural bias that makes us think, *I should be able to fix this myself, so I'll use the chemicals that I have available to me to do that.*

Basically, you are using depressants to treat your disease. Numbing or masking serious symptoms to your lifelong condition will only make it worse.

Don't underestimate the negative effects of alcohol and drugs on your mind and body. Why do we abuse illegal drugs and alcohol when we have some of the strongest pharmaceutical drugs at our disposal? The right medications can give you a daily high. It's not necessary to give up drinking or partying completely; just find balance.

Take the responsibility to not abuse alcohol or drugs and to go from drinking or partying too much to not too much. Too much is detrimental to your mind and body.

Ruth gives the following advice:

> I love to smoke pot and drink tequila like it is going out of style. My problem is I abuse them. I get high as a kite, drink too much, and have a hangover the next day that hurts all day long. These days, I still smoke a joint now and then and drink some Cuervo, but I use them in moderation and don't abuse them. Instead, I use my medications to make me feel good, and the best part, it's legal, unlike pot. I don't risk getting arrested or feeling like crap all day long because I drank too much. In fact, I believe my medications give me more mental and physical prowess than many people who are not bipolar. I have been taking the same meds for two years and I know I am at the top of my game.

Dial In Your Medications

Dialing in your medications to the optimal dosage is one of the most important skills to master. This is where the rubber meets the road. Most bipolar individuals take more than one medicine at a time, and determining the "medication cocktail" that works takes time, patience, and skill. It's important to work closely with your psychiatrist and reevaluate your medication regularly, as the optimum dose may change over time. Self-reflection and writing in a journal can also help you keep track of the way your mood shifts from day to day.

In order to dial in the optimal dosages of your medications, you must become proficient at researching the medicine, rating your medications, ramping up the medicine, ramping down the medicine, and mixing the perfect medication cocktail.

Researching the Medicine

Being aware of the pros and cons of any new prescription is a must for dialing in your medication to the optimal dosage. Research each medication you take using online resources, the expertise of your psychiatrist, and talking to other bipolar people who are taking the same medication. Find out the answers to the following questions:

- How will I know if the medicine is working?
- What are the expected results (pros) of the medicine?
- What are the side effects and risks (cons) of the medicine?
- What is the target dosage (therapeutic range) for this medication?
- What dosage of this medicine do most patients take?
- What time of day should I take the medicine?
- Are there any foods or other substances I will need to avoid?
- How will this drug interact with my other prescriptions?

Rating Your Medications

It is very helpful to have a methodology to use to determine if your medicine is dialed in to the optimum dosage. Answer the following questions to rate how well your medicine is working:

- Are you sleeping well?
- Are your moods generally positive?

- Does the medicine provide benefits?
- Do you have any bipolar symptoms?
- How is your energy level?
- Do you have any side effects?
- Do you have a romantic partner and/or friends you socialize with?
- Do you feel good physically?
- Are you thinking clearly?
- What does your heart tell you?
- Do you have sexual awareness and drive?
- Do you feel stable?
- Do you feel angry?
- Do you feel like a robot?
- Are you overly anxious?
- Are you depressed?
- Are you manic?

Ramping Up the Medicine

The beginning stage of dialing in the medication is the ramp-up stage, in which you start with a low dosage and increase it until you reach the "therapeutic range." The therapeutic range is where the level of medicine (drug) in the blood is great enough to provide the required therapeutic response but small enough to restrict the possibility of side effects. Learning how to ramp up a medicine to the optimum dosage is a skill that will serve you well the rest of your life.

Ruth describes dialing in a medication called Lamictal.

> The reason I started taking Lamictal for treating my bipolar illness is because my psychiatrist told me one of the foremost experts on bipolar disorder in the U.S. claims the best medicine combination for

treating bipolar disorder is Lithium and Lamictal. My psychiatrist told me his patients take a range of dosage of Lamictal from 200 milligrams to 700 milligrams a day. He warned me that a very serious side effect to watch out for is a rash. He told me if I get a rash to discontinue taking Lamictal immediately because it could actually kill me. His instructions for ramping up the medicine was to start at 100 milligrams for a week, then advance to 200 milligrams, and continue increasing by 100 milligrams every week until I judged the medication was working optimally. He instructed me to not go over a dosage of 400 milligrams a day until we talked again. I am currently taking 400 milligrams a day and feel great, have lots of energy, and a positive attitude.

Ramping Down the Medicine

You have to be smart enough to know when you have given a medicine a fair chance and when it is time to try a different medicine. This is totally your decision: If it doesn't work, it doesn't work. You will know as long as you are keeping a watchful eye. If you decide you are going to stop taking a particular medicine, then it is a very bad idea to stop taking it all at once. Without ramping down your medications, you risk skyrocketing into mania or cliff diving into depression.

Psychiatric medications are extremely powerful, and it takes your mind time to adjust. That is why it is so important to ramp down the dosage of particular medications. A good number of episodes could be avoided if people weaned themselves slowly off the medicine in a controlled fashion instead of deciding to stop taking their medicines cold turkey. Even if you wean yourself off the medicine in a controlled fashion, it is still going to be a challenge. It will take time for your mind to adjust, so count on some unpleasantness and be prepared to ride out uncomfortable feelings and sensations until the medicine is out of your system completely.

If one of your medicines does not work for you, meet with your psychiatrist as soon as you can to figure out the next step to take. Since that medicine didn't work, talk with your doctor about what other medications he or she recommends.

The Perfect Medication Cocktail

You may have to try a number of different medicines before you zero in on the right medication cocktail. Keep in mind that the pharmaceutical-grade medicines used to treat bipolar disorder are extremely powerful and that each medicine has its own effects and reactions with other medicines. Finding the right combination and dosages of medicines to effectively treat your bipolar disorder is a trial-and-error process that can take weeks or months. The cocktail is different for every individual. For you to attain peace of mind, optimal brain functioning, good energy levels, and overall well-being, you have to keep experimenting with different medicine combinations until the results meet or exceed your expectations and criteria.

Just getting by is not good enough; settling for less than happiness is a cop-out. Life is short. The right combination of medicines can make you strong, happy, and whole again. Your heart will know when you have found the "Holy Grail" of medicines that make you glad you are alive!

As time goes by and you experiment with different medicines, you will become more proficient at dialing in the medications to the optimum dosages for treating your disease. If all indications are that the medicine or medicine combination is a go, congratulations! You have successfully dialed in your medication.

Beware of Side Effects!

Any time you start taking a new medication, you must be on the lookout for side effects. A side effect is any unwanted, nontherapeutic effect caused by a drug. Most psychiatric medicines have side effects of one kind or another. Some people are prone to experience side effects from a particular medicine, while others do not experience any side effects from the same medicine. It is extremely important to watch out for side effects. Be wary because some side effects are more serious than others. *Some can actually kill you!* Any psychiatrist worth his or her salt will inform you of the possible side effects when prescribing medication. If he or she doesn't warn you of the possible side effects of the medicine, then get a new psychiatrist.

Side effects lie in wait like a lion stalking its prey until the medicine reaches a certain threshold in your bloodstream. Side effects may happen quickly or may occur several days after you begin taking the medicine; some may not show up until much later, when you have increased the dosage to a certain level. *Take heed because this could be weeks or months after you start taking the medication.* Everything may be going along smoothly, and then BAM! Things turn bad—and very quickly.

If something is going wrong physically or mentally, always look to the medicine as the possible culprit. The following examples describe extremely undesirable side effects that two individuals experienced due to two medicines: Risperdal and Wellbutrin.

These particular scenarios should not turn you off of the idea of trying one of these medications since everyone is affected differently.

Gary started taking Risperdal in place of a medicine he had been taking called Neurontin because he didn't think Neurontin was beneficial. He started taking 2 milligrams a day of Risperdal for two weeks, upped it to 4 milligrams for two more weeks, and then increased it to 5 milligrams and stabilized at this dosage. Risperdal definitely was beneficial. He had good energy, concentration and a good mental attitude, so Gary made the decision to stay on it. Everything was going great for eight weeks or so, until one night he and his wife started fooling around and he didn't get aroused. He and his wife hadn't been getting along so he thought that was the cause. This went on for several weeks, and Gary didn't attribute it to the medicine since he had been taking the same dosage for the last two months. Just like any other guy would feel, Gary knew this was serious business and totally unacceptable. He ordered some Viagra over the counter from Canada and finally got back into action. During his next scheduled visit with his psychiatrist, Gary told him what was going on. His doctor pulled out a medicine reference book about six inches thick and looked up Risperdal. He told Gary that the percentage of people who suffer the side effect of impotence due to Risperdal was up to 13 percent. Gary told his psychiatrist, "I'm going off this fucking medicine." After he got off the Risperdal, he no longer needed the Viagra.

Jane began taking a medicine called Wellbutrin to help her bipolar illness. After three days, she began vomiting almost instantaneously, without any warning. She puked inside her car and on her living room rug. She couldn't act quickly enough to stop the car or make it to the bathroom. She thought she had the stomach flu. A couple of days later, still puking out of the blue, she attributed it to the medicine and made an appointment with her psychiatrist. The doctor told her it was more than likely the Wellbutrin. He told her that up to 20 percent of people who take Wellbutrin experience the side effect of puking. Jane discontinued the medication and thought, *Why didn't this dipshit psychiatrist tell me about the possible side effects?"* She decided to find a new psychiatrist.

You may be taking more than one medicine at the same time and are not sure which medicine is causing the side effect. Very likely the side effect is a result of the most recent medicine you added to your regime or a change (increase) in the dosage of a medication. However, this is not always the case. Either way, take immediate action if something strange or unusual is going on, mentally or physically.

Some medicines have side effects that will taper off as your body gets used to the dosage level. For example, you may feel dizzy when you reach a certain dosage, but the dizziness goes away once you take that dosage for a few days. You will have to judge the seriousness of the side effect. If it is tolerable, see if the side effect subsides after a day or two.

The bottom line is that you must monitor yourself mentally and physically when you are taking any kind of medication. If anything unusual starts happening, immediately call your doctor and get an appointment.

A list of generic side effects to watch out for when taking medication for bipolar disorder follows:

Generic Side Effects from Bipolar Medications

- severe anxiety
- sedation
- insomnia
- sexual dysfunction
- tremor
- excessive thirst/dry mouth
- increased urination
- stomach pain
- agitation
- muscle stiffness/pain
- loss of coordination
- vomiting
- weight gain/increased appetite
- hallucinations
- weight loss
- drowsiness
- constipation
- blackouts
- rashes or itching
- sensitivity to the sun
- headaches

Medicine Noncompliance

Caution: *The top risk factor for relapse into a bipolar episode is going off your meds.*

Jane tells about her challenges with bipolar medications.

I resisted taking medication for a number of years after my first bipolar episode. I would take if for a while but a few months later get disgruntled that it wasn't working and I was wasting my life away. I felt like a robot with no real feelings. There were probably a couple of episodes that wouldn't have ended up so badly except I went off my medicine. My most recent episode (three years ago) began a week after I stopped taking Lithium. I ended up heavily medicated in a psychiatric hospital for several days. I accepted I need medication to avoid future episodes, and I have been taking my medication on a daily basis and have not had an episode since.

There are several reasons that we stop taking our medication.

- We don't think the medication is helping.
- The medicine causes side effects.
- We plan to start taking medicine again if we experience any bipolar symptoms.
- A manic episode begins and our thoughts go wild. We love the highs of being manic. *I don't need any stinking medicine!* we think.
- We want to be "ourselves."
- We think we are smarter now that we have experienced an episode and can use our willpower to keep from having another episode.

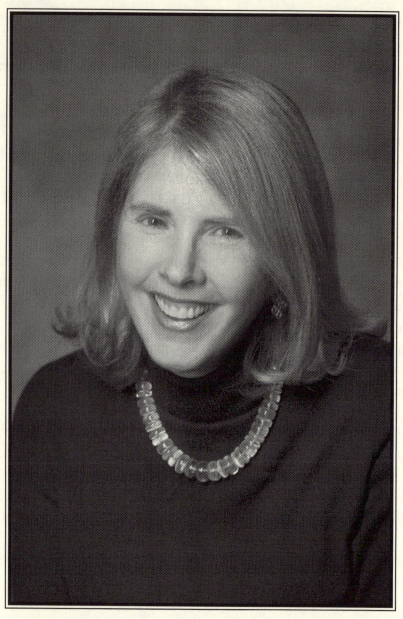

No pill can help me deal with the problem of not wanting to take pills; likewise, no amount of psychotherapy alone can prevent my manias and depressions. I need both.
—Kay Jamison, professor of psychiatry, writer

CHAPTER 5
Choose the Right Psychiatrist

There are good and bad psychiatrists, just as there are good and bad professionals in any trade or industry. The skills, abilities, and competence of your psychiatrist to repair, tune up, and maintain your mind can be likened to that of a trusted auto mechanic who is the only person you let work on your car. Finding a good psychiatrist who is right for you can seem like a long, involved process; however, knowing that this doctor is the one you are trusting to treat your bipolar illness and keep you healthy and sane (and alive), as well as possibly partner with you for a lifetime, makes it well worth your time and effort.

Choosing a good psychiatrist is crucial to managing your illness and can be a powerful weapon in the war with bipolar disorder. A psychiatrist is a medical doctor who works to prevent, diagnose and treat mental, emotional, and behavioral problems. A psychiatrist's medical training allows him to order medical tests and prescribe medication as well as provide psychotherapy (talk therapy). Psychiatrists complete four years of medical school plus four years in a psychiatric residency program. Their education requires time spent in classrooms, medical offices, and hospitals, working directly with patients and other medical professionals. These are well-educated people devoted to helping others. But, again, not all psychiatrists are the same.

Choosing a psychiatrist is no easy feat because someone else's "good" may not be good for you. The best course of action is to research and interview a doctor—just like hiring any other employee. While "good" is different for each person, one thing remains the same: a good psychiatrist is one with whom you are happy. That's all. A good psychiatrist is one who performs to your expectations, whatever those are.

Trust is by far the most important aspect to consider when choosing a psychiatrist. You are putting your trust in this person with your emotional and physical well-being. This is your life. The most important aspect of your psychiatrist's role is to be available anytime, day or night, in your time of crisis. A psychiatrist needs to get back to you in a hurry if you call for help. If you need help quickly, tell the secretary or after-hours doctor on call that you need someone to contact you immediately.

Scott tells about an episode that most likely would not have spiraled into disaster if his psychiatrist had only answered his call for help.

> I started having serious symptoms that were very similar to my previous manic episodes and recognized I needed help. I called my psychiatrist's office at ten a.m. and told the receptionist it was urgent that I get an appointment. She said he was booked all day today and tomorrow, but he had an opening on Wednesday at nine a.m. I told her

I needed to talk to him today as soon as possible. She said she would give him the message. He never called and, two days later, when the secretary called back to remind me of my appointment, I was too far gone to keep the appointment. I was manic as manic can be. This episode could have been avoided and I probably wouldn't have ended up in the psychiatric hospital if the doctor had called me back within a few hours of my call for help. I found another psychiatrist once I recovered.

Rating a Psychiatrist

Here are a number of criteria for finding a good psychiatrist:

- He establishes a contingency plan with you and tells you to call day or night if you need help.
- He gives you instructions on how to modify your medication in the event of bipolar symptoms.
- He is skillful at determining your state of mind and zeroing in on your current problems.
- You feel like you can trust him.
- He is easy to talk to, and you have good rapport.
- He has several years of experience treating bipolar disorder.
- He has hands-on experience in psychiatric hospitals.
- He provides psychotherapy (self-talk).
- He promotes a whole-life wellness plan.
- He is extremely knowledgeable about medication.
- He explains the pros and cons of medicine, including possible side effects.
- He explains how to ramp up the medicine to the therapeutic range.

- He has common sense and gives good advice.
- He is covered by your insurance.
- He is located at a convenient location.
- He won't put up with bullshit.
- He is knowledgeable about newly developed methods for treating bipolar disorder.
- He is board certified.
- He listens to your questions and doesn't interrupt or judge you.
- He sees you within a reasonable amount of time of your appointment time.
- He explains the meaning of difficult terms and communicates effectively with you.
- He is affiliated with a hospital that's important to you.

Psychotherapy (Talk Therapy)

Besides prescribing medication, many psychiatrists provide psychotherapy, or "talk" therapy. Therapy helps people reduce stress, regulate moods, and change thinking patterns that may trigger episodes. Also, research has established that using "talk therapy" in combination with medication to treat bipolar disorder further reduces both the number of relapses that people experience and the severity of those relapses. One of the most important outcomes of therapy is self-awareness. For a person with bipolar disorder, self-awareness may mean things like realizing the different events that are likely to trigger a relapse and recognizing the signs and symptoms of the onset of depression or mania.

In her book *Touched with Fire,* Kay Jamison discusses the benefits of psychotherapy.

Psychotherapy, in conjunction with medication, is often essential to healing as well as to the prevention of possible recurrences. Drug therapy, which is primary, frees most patients from the severe disruptions of manic and depressive episodes. Psychotherapy can help individuals come to terms with the repercussions of past episodes, take the medications that are necessary to prevent recurrence, and better understand and deal with the often devastating psychological implications and consequences of having manic-depressive illness. (Jamison 1994, 17)

Finding a New Psychiatrist

Here are some helpful pointers to finding a new psychiatrist.

- If you have insurance and want to stay in the network, call your insurance company for a list of names.
- If you know someone who likes his or her doctor, see that doctor.
- If you know someone who likes his or her doctor but you can't see that specific doctor, ask your friend to get some names of other psychiatrists or call the doctor yourself.
- Call your state psychiatric society and ask for a referral.
- Ask your primary care doctor. He or she is used to making referrals.
- Ask *any* psychiatrist. They tend to know one another. If you can get one on the phone, he or she may give you names even without seeing you in person.

- If you're a student, try the school's counseling or health center. The staff there may also be able to suggest off-campus referrals.
- Search online and query listservs, LinkedIn, Facebook, and other social media sites. Pick a few out of the heap and research them. The easiest way do this is through websites such as HealthGrades.com, which allows you to find doctors by name, specialty, and location. But what's better is that it provides feedback on the doctors, including a background check, which is excellent information to have before you walk into a doctor's office.

No-Cost Initial Appointments

Once you have found a potential psychiatrist, call and make an appointment. Explain what you want help for when you call and ask if they are taking new patients. If so, ask if you can schedule a no-cost initial meeting.

For your first appointment, you need to decide what to ask the doctor to find out if he's a good fit for you. During the first meeting, the doctor is going to be interviewing you. But remember that you are the client and should be interviewing him or her as well. What you ask depends on what you care about in a doctor and in your treatment.

These questions are about opening a dialogue on issues that matter to you. It's not about judgment as much as it is about exploration. You're testing the waters to see if this is the person you think is most able to help you. Do not be intimidated by them whatsoever just because they are doctors.

Here are some questions you may wish to ask:

- How long have you been practicing as a psychiatrist?
- What percentage of your patients are bipolar?
- What happens if I have an emergency outside of office hours?
- Have you ever worked in a psychiatric ward or hospital?
- What is your treatment philosophy?
- What is your view on bipolar disorder and psychotherapy?
- How often do you typically see your patients?
- How long are appointments?
- What medications do you typically prescribe for your bipolar patients?
- What is your view on supplements and alternative medication?
- Are there any medical conditions that could be causing or exacerbating my mood swings?

It is okay if a doctor doesn't meet your expectations. Not every doctor is for every person, and there's nothing necessarily wrong with either of you. If it doesn't work, it doesn't work. It's like a first date. First dates don't always lead to second dates. If you decide it is not going to be a good match, now is the easiest time to say something simple like, "I don't think we're the best therapeutic match. Could you please provide a referral to someone else?"

Scott describes his search for a psychiatrist.

> It took me awhile to find a psychiatrist who I felt I could trust to save my life if need be, prescribe the best medicines for me, and help me overcome my

bipolar illness. I had no-cost initial meetings with three psychiatrists and interviewed them to decide if I wanted a long-term relationship with them. The third one I met impressed me and I have been with her for the past three years episode free.

Ultimately, at the end of the day, it is your life, and who to hire to be your psychiatrist is your choice. Your psychiatrist works for you. He or she is your employee, and you pay her or him for services. You decide whether to hire or fire him or her.

Getting the Most Out of Appointments

Prior to having an appointment with your psychiatrist, prepare in advance what you want to discuss and accomplish. When the appointment begins, the psychiatrist will try to gauge how you are doing and your state of mind. If you are manic, depressed, or experiencing noticeable bipolar symptoms, tell your doctor.

After questioning you about your mood and state of mind, your psychiatrist will ascertain what dosage you are taking of each of your medications. Then he will assess your medication regimen and decide, based on your input, whether to increase or decrease a dosage and perhaps counsel you to go off a medicine or to start a new one. Before the appointment, decide whether you are happy with your medications or feel that a change is needed. If the medicine is not working, try to figure out the reason why. Keeping a log is very helpful. The more specific you can be, the better your doctor can counsel you. Other factors to discuss at your appointment are how things are going overall with your physical health, relationships, and career.

Ruth relates how she prepared for a recent appointment with her psychiatrist.

> A few days before my regularly scheduled three-month appointment with my doctor, I considered how things were going in my life. I reviewed my mental state, energy level, relationships, last time I got laid (too long), and how my job and career were going. My conclusion was I was too much of a wimp. I wasn't meeting any guys, although I'm fairly attractive. In general, I wasn't pleased with my personality, being too laid back and not very sociable. The positives were that I was focused, loved my job, and was in good physical health. I asked him what changes I could make with my medications to be more assertive. He told me to decrease the dosage I was taking of Depakote from 750 milligrams to 500 milligrams.

Your psychiatrist is not in charge of what medications you take. You are! The doctor prescribes medication for you and then will make modifications based upon your feedback. It is your responsibility to keep making changes to your medications until you find the right recipe that keeps you balanced. It's your life, your brain, and your happiness that are at stake. Keep working with your psychiatrist, monitoring yourself, educating yourself, and making adjustments to your medications until you are happy with the results.

These are some typical questions a psychiatrist might ask during an appointment.

- How's your mood?
- How's your job?
- Have you been exercising?

- How's your diet?
- Do you take vitamin supplements like fish oil, vitamin B, and vitamin D?
- Are you dating anyone?
- How's your relationship with your kids, family, and friends?

Besides prescribing medication, a psychiatrist is usually (but not always) responsible for therapy. The only way for a psychiatrist or counselor to help is for you to be brutally honest with him and yourself. Tell him about any bipolar symptoms you are having and what you are thinking and feeling.

Jane conveys a conversation she had with her psychiatrist.

> I told my psychiatrist that I was unsure about my relationship with Murray, who had moved in with me six months ago. We have fun together and great sex, but we fight a lot unless we have a few drinks. My psychiatrist advised me to quit drinking with Murray and see how we get along. It took me a while to cool it on the drinking, but I came across two people I respected who had quit drinking in the last couple of years. Talking with them convinced me to give up drinking for awhile because I wanted clarity on my relationship with Murray. After I had quit drinking for two months, we decided to split up. Murray said I wasn't fun anymore, and we really didn't have much in common. He moved out and I am much happier.

When to Get a New Psychiatrist

You will know if you are not happy with your psychiatrist in general. Make sure it's not just because you are in a bad mood that week or have taken offense at something he said. Don't continue to stagnate with the same psychiatrist if you are not seeing any benefit.

If you decide to move on, don't burn bridges with your current psychiatrist until you have found another psychiatrist whom you trust to prescribe your medication. This is important because you don't want to be at a disadvantage when interviewing a possible new psychiatrist because you need him to write you prescriptions right away.

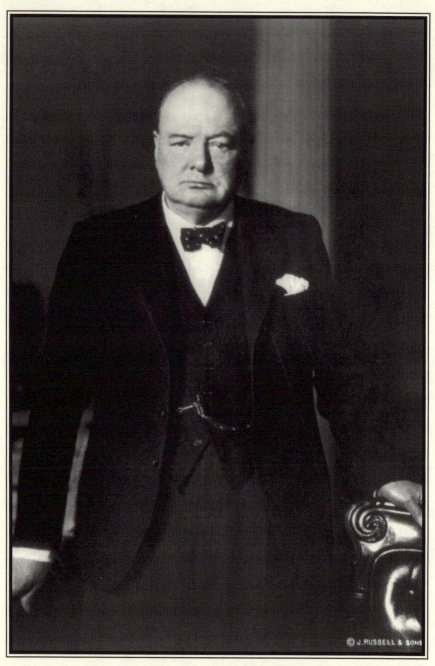

If you're going through hell, keep going.
—Winston Churchill, prime minister

CHAPTER 6
Stalk the Enemy

There is no cure for bipolar disorder, only treatment and management. The more you learn about bipolar illness, the better you will be able to prepare yourself for the battles ahead. Learning to manage and eliminate symptoms has everything to do with self-knowledge. Once you learn the patterns of bipolar disorder and specific strategies to treat the mood swings and their symptoms, you can learn to live with the illness and achieve what you want from life.

"This Murderous Cauldron"

> In a rage I pulled the bathroom lamp off the wall. I see in the mirror blood running down my arms, collecting into the tight ribbing of my beautiful, erotic negligee, only an hour ago used in passion of an altogether different and wonderful kind. I can't help it, I chant to myself, but I can't say it; the words won't come out, and the thoughts are going by far too fast. I bang my head over and over against the door. God, make it stop, I can't stand it. I know I'm insane again. I can't think, I can't calm this murderous cauldron, my grand ideas of an hour ago seem absurd and pathetic, my

life is in ruins, and—worse still—ruinous; my body is uninhabitable. It is raging and weeping and full of destruction and wild energy gone amok. In the mirror I see a creature I don't know but must live and share my mind with. I understand why Jekyll killed himself before Hyde had taken over completely; I took a massive overdose of Lithium with no regrets. (Jamison 1996, 113)

The above excerpt from the book *An Unquiet Mind* by Kay Jamison illustrates the changes in mood that intensify as a bipolar episode progresses. Kay goes from having "grand ideas" to an hour later feeling like she is "insane again" and her body is "uninhabitable." When a bipolar episode has progressed to this state, there is nothing that can stop you from crashing and burning other than being heavily sedated with medication. Fortunately, Kay Jamison was rescued from this suicide attempt and continues her career as a professor of psychiatry at the Johns Hopkins University School of Medicine, as well as a renowned author of books on mental illness.

What Is Bipolar Disorder?

Bipolar disorder is a chronic illness that is best described as a mood disorder. This mental illness causes unusual and dramatic shifts in mood, energy, and the ability to think clearly. The mood of someone who is bipolar rotates between polar opposites: at one end of the spectrum is highs (manic) and at the other end is lows. The most identifiable bipolar symptoms are these polar mood swings, each of which can last anywhere from days to weeks. Not everyone's symptoms are the same, and the severity of mania and depression can vary. Some people have "mixed states" in which they feel both mania and depression at the same time.

Bipolar disorder can affect a person's energy level, judgment, memory, concentration, appetite, sleep patterns, sex drive, and self-esteem. Bipolar disorder has also been linked to anxiety, substance abuse, and health problems such as diabetes, heart disease, migraines, and high blood pressure. You may be asking yourself, *What doesn't bipolar affect?*

Some people alternate between extreme episodes of mania and depression, but most are depressed more often than they are manic. People with bipolar disorder may also go for long stretches without symptoms. However, the condition is usually cyclical, so be prepared for it to worsen and then improve at times. For those of us who live with bipolar disorder, this means accepting that mood swings and episodes of mania or depression will always be a potential challenge for us.

My dad was bipolar in the extreme but never admitted it or took medicine to control it. He would become manic and be high as a kite for several weeks, usually heading to Las Vegas or Atlantic City to gamble heavily. During his manic periods, he was busy: managing his bar business, playing poker, attempting to start other businesses and enjoying life. He would talk to us kids and be involved with our lives, much more so than when he was depressed. The times when he was depressed were far worse. When he came down from a manic episode, he would sit in his La-Z-Boy watching television in his robe, day after day, week after week, uncommunicative and down in the dumps. He kept the bar running from his La-Z-Boy, and the only other thing he paid attention to was the television. These depressed periods of time were much longer than the manic periods of time. Having witnessed the detrimental effects of bipolar disorder on my dad I vowed not to let bipolar disorder beat me down like it did him.

Mania

Remember this rule of thumb if you are experiencing a manic episode: "What goes up must come down." Mania causes people with bipolar illness to climb higher and higher and then crash like a wave rolling into the shore.

When experiencing mania, the bipolar individual is very productive, running around like there is never enough to do. They tend to be really happy and optimistic about life. If a person has extreme manic episodes, hallucinations and psychotic symptoms are possible. Psychosis is a state in which a person is unable to tell the difference between reality and non-reality. Psychotic symptoms include hallucinations and false beliefs about having special powers or a special identity (such as believing you are God, have superhuman strength, or have X-ray vision). This can be a really cool experience, with the mind offering escape, but it is not reality.

During a manic episode, a person might impulsively quit a job, charge up huge amounts on credit cards, or feel rested after sleeping only two hours. Manic symptoms can include minute-to-minute mood swings, rapid speech, grandiosity, impulsiveness, delusions, the feeling of complete invincibility, and the absolute conviction that certain untrue things are true. A manic state can be identified by feelings of extreme euphoria or irritability, agitation, surges of energy, a reduced need for sleep, talkativeness, pleasure seeking, and increased risk-taking behavior.

Another manic symptom called psychomotor agitation exists when someone experiences unintentional purposeless physical activities that arise from tension and anxiety. They may pace around a room, wring their hands, or more dangerous motions such as ripping, tearing, or chewing at the skin around the mouth.

Depression

When most people think of bipolar disorder, they think of the manic side. However, depression is the far more common and more damaging of the two poles. In the euphoria of mania, people rarely choose to intentionally harm themselves. In a deep depression, however, self-mutilation and suicidal thoughts and actions are far too common.

Depression is a form of reversible brain failure. When someone is depressed, it's like his or her computer's central processing unit (CPU) isn't working properly. As a result, focusing on anything is very difficult. Depression fills one with negative thoughts, almost like an intrusion. When depressed, individuals with bipolar illness may stay in bed all day, feeling that they cannot get going.

Depressive symptoms may include dreariness, extreme pessimism, hopelessness, and lack of focus. People with bipolar illness may feel that their thoughts move slowly, and they take little pleasure in any activity. Bipolar individuals in a depressed phase often feel as if they are worthless and that their lives are meaningless. They often isolate themselves from others. They may begin to overeat and, given their low activity level, gain weight. They may speak or think of suicide or become violent, making emergency care crucial for their safety. Just as they do in manic episodes, psychotic symptoms may occur during severe depressive episodes.

People who are depressed undergo a series of physical and emotional changes. They can experience fatigue, as well as a symptom called psychomotor retardation. Psychomotor retardation slows down a person's ability to process information, thereby impairing concentration on work or other tasks. It also slows down physical movements, speech, and thought processes.

Mixed Episode

This is a mood episode during which the symptoms of depression and mania are experienced at the same time. This can lead to irritability, hostility, and physical aggression. Depending on the severity of the symptoms, patients are hospitalized for their safety and the safety of those around them. They may need a longer hospital stay or a combination of more than one medication to get well.

Seasonal Pattern

Seasonal pattern describes mood disorders that are triggered by a particular season of the year. For example, someone who tends to become manic during the spring and summer and then returns to a regular mood during the late fall and winter has a seasonal pattern of mania. Alternatively, someone who tends to become depressed during the late fall and winter and then returns to a regular mood during the spring and summer has a seasonal pattern of depression. "The fall/winter depression pattern is more common than the spring/summer pattern. Suicide is far more common in March, April and May, probably due to changes in light" (Martin 2006).

Each bipolar individual has his or her own specific footprint of mania and depression. Pay attention to your moods during different seasons of the year and determine if you have a seasonal mood pattern. If so, you can adjust your treatment plan accordingly.

Bipolar Episode Triggers

"Triggers" are outside events that can set off new episodes of mania or depression or make existing bipolar symptoms worse. Triggers are the main environmental causes of bipolar disorder mood swings and must be monitored and reduced as much as possible. One of the best ways to prevent future episodes is identifying and avoiding the specific triggers that ignite your bipolar symptoms. Lack of sleep, going off of your medications, and major stress are three of the top triggers of relapse into a bipolar episode.

Scott tells about two bipolar triggers he has learned to avoid.

> I used to get stressed out whenever I traveled back to Ohio for family gatherings at my mom and dad's. A couple of years ago, I came back from a visit for a week over the Christmas holidays and ended up having a bipolar episode and being depressed for a couple of months. I figured out that the two biggest stress factors for me during these visits are being around a large group of people and not having my own place to retreat. I still go home to visit but not

during the holidays. I go when I can visit with just a few people at a time. Also, I stay in a hotel instead of staying at my mom and dad's place. Since I made these two changes, my last two visits have been good.

For each of us, our stressors and triggers are different. Identifying the triggers that may set you off beforehand can help you to avoid an episode. Once you identify your personal triggers, you can work on recognizing them as they occur and handling them more effectively. A list of triggers should include a list of those things from past episodes that were occurring when your episode started.

Common triggers of bipolar episodes include the following:

- sleep irregularities
- financial problems
- increase in stress
- isolation
- going off medications
- alcohol or drug abuse
- medicinal side effects
- change of seasons
- forgetting to take medicine
- conflict with others
- new relationships
- lack of exercise
- birth of a child
- travel/jet lag
- feelings of loneliness and despair
- nonsupportive family/friends
- relationship breakups/problems
- change in smoking habits

- a death in the family
- stress at work
- promotion at work
- a vacation
- change in environment
- moving residences
- poor nutrition
- physical illness
- loss of employment
- taking on more than you can handle
- changing jobs
- thyroid malfunction

Sleep Disturbances

Sleep disturbances are a key symptom of both mania and depression *and* an excellent early warning sign of a mood change. Bipolar disorder is highly influenced by the circadian system, which is the body's twenty-four-hour internal biological clock. The circadian rhythm of your body determines when you need sleep and when you need to wake. It is through this rhythm that your body knows when to start and stop certain chemicals in your brain. To put it simply, regulated sleep stabilizes the brain chemicals that control emotions. Maintaining a consistent sleep schedule and wake time can help you avoid nighttime sleeplessness or daytime exhaustion, which can increase the risk of new episodes of mania or depression.

Regulating sleep is often one of the best ways to balance moods and the circadian system. When you go to sleep easily, sleep and dream deeply, and then wake up refreshed on a set schedule every day, you're experiencing regulated sleep.

Unfortunately, maintaining a regular sleep schedule is not always as easy as it sounds, especially if your neighbors, family, roommates, schedule, lifestyle, or sleeping arrangements do not cooperate. The more you upset the natural circadian rhythm by working odd hours, staying out late and partying, ignoring what you put into your body, or watching upsetting television before bedtime, the less likely you are to find stability. You may need to change some of these behaviors in order to kick your circadian rhythm into gear so that you can sleep better and give your brain and your body time to recharge. Sticking to a sleep routine, winding down with pre-bedtime rituals, reducing caffeine intake, and getting your family or roommates to cooperate are very helpful.

These are some common contributors to unregulated sleep.

- shift work or work that upsets your sleep patterns such as an ever-changing schedule
- stress
- drugs and alcohol
- caffeine
- travel to different time zones
- anything new: new baby, new job, loss of a job, new city, etc.
- frisky bed partner
- bright light before bed

Learn to avoid the events and circumstances that may trigger you to have a bipolar episode. If something triggers you into sliding into an episode, launch your contingency plan ASAP. Don't let something trigger you into having a catastrophic episode that could cause you to do something harmful or detrimental to yourself or your life.

Bipolar Disorder Is Predictable

What is your bipolar modus operandi? Bipolar disorder can look very different in different people. The symptoms vary widely in their pattern, severity, and frequency. Some people are more prone to either mania or depression, while others alternate equally between the two poles. Some have frequent mood disruptions, while others experience only a few over a lifetime.

However, bipolar disorder is somewhat predictable. For each person, the disorder tends to follow a pattern. It has some consistency. Within the broad groupings of manic and depressive symptoms, each person will have his or her own "markers," or unique expressions of the illness that help to define that person's personal brand of bipolar disorder. For example, you may notice racing speech and thoughts, prolonged periods of irritability or anger, decreased need for sleep, or delusions of grandeur. Recognizing that you are having similar symptoms to ones you experienced during past bipolar episodes can be a *huge advantage* if you are able to take evasive action (launch your contingency plan) sooner rather than later.

As you become familiar with your illness, you can learn your own unique patterns of behavior. If you learn to recognize these signs and seek effective and timely care, you can often prevent additional episodes. Recognizing and naming your typical bipolar episode symptoms is the first important step to understanding and beginning to take control over your bipolar disease.

Gary describes the symptoms he experienced at the onset of his past bipolar episodes.

> At the beginning of my bipolar episodes, I become more expansive, seem more in tune with other people, and don't sleep as much. A common symptom seems to be attributing hidden meanings to everything that happens. For example, I attribute hidden meanings to what people say, even if they are not talking to me, as omens. Another symptom I experience is hearing God talking directly to me telling me what to do. These days I try to keep tabs on what I am thinking and monitor my mood on a regular basis. If I notice any of these symptoms I know I better do something fast because an episode is brewing.

Scott has also learned to monitor himself closely for bipolar symptoms based on previous episodes.

> My bipolar episodes always begin on the manic side. There is a critical juncture in time where I realize that I am having off-the-wall thoughts, or other symptoms, and I know I need help. At this point in time, I usually make an attempt to get help by calling my psychiatrist. However, if I don't talk to him or see him within an hour or two of the call, it's too late, game over. I become more and more obstinate. My mania grows exponentially and my episode becomes like a runaway freight train without any brakes.

Bipolar Disorder Facts and Statistics

The following facts and statistics characterize the true nature of bipolar illness.

Note: The numbers and statistics presented here are representative of research from a number of sources, including both online and published material.

- The percentage of bipolar patients who have attempted suicide is 25 percent to 50 percent (Caruso 2009).
- The percentage of bipolar patients whose suicide attempts have resulted in death: 15 percent to 20 percent. This is the highest suicide rate of any psychiatric disorder (Novick and Swartz 2010).
- Lack of sleep, going off of medications, and major stress are three of the top causes of relapse into a bipolar episode.
- About 40 percent of people with bipolar disorder struggle with alcohol and drug abuse (Evans 2000).
- A large percentage of people with bipolar illness go off of their medication due to side effects, the desire for manic energy, or impaired insight.
- In the euphoria of mania, people rarely choose to intentionally harm themselves. In a deep depression, however, self-mutilation and suicidal thoughts and actions are common.
- A powerful combination to fight bipolar illness is to create a whole-life wellness plan that includes a simple diet, therapeutic techniques, and plenty of exercise, as well as taking regular medications.

- Bipolar disorder affects approximately 5.7 million American adults, or about 2.6 percent of the US population age eighteen and older in a given year (Kessler 2005).
- Life expectancy of an adult with bipolar disorder is approximately fifteen years shorter than that of a person without (Cowen 2011).
- Approximately 25 percent of bipolar individuals are obese (McElroy 2002).
- People with bipolar disorder are three times more likely to develop diabetes than members of the general population (Thompson 2010).
- Sleep disturbances are a key symptom of both mania and depression *and* an excellent early warning sign of a mood change.
- Three of the top methods of bipolar suicide are guns, suffocation (hanging), and poisoning (overdose) (Mariant 2012).
- Approximately 15 percent of people with bipolar disorder have had a violent episode. Bipolar individuals are prone to agitation that may result in impulsive aggression (as opposed to premeditated aggression) during manic and mixed episodes. However, depressed states, which can involve intense agitation and irritability, also carry a risk of violent behavior (Vann 2010).
- Bipolar disorder doesn't discriminate by age, race, ethnicity, or social class. It affects as many men as women (Sachs 2008).
- At this time, bipolar disorder is not curable.
- Knowing and accepting that you have bipolar disorder can be healing. Self-awareness of your bipolar illness can effectively protect you from severe or life-threatening events. If you know you have this

condition, then you are in a better position to protect your life, your family, and your career.
- Many diseases can be detected by some kind of medical test—for example, blood tests for diabetes and kidney function or CT scans for brain tumors. This is not the case for bipolar disorder. Unfortunately, there is not a test that can determine whether you are bipolar.
- Bipolar disorder is often hereditary and tends to run in families. A person with the disorder most likely has a parent or relative who is bipolar.

Causes of Bipolar Disorder

The exact cause of bipolar disorder is unknown. It is not clear whether it may lie dormant in the brain and be activated on its own or it may be triggered by environmental factors such as social circumstances, psychological stress, abuse, significant loss, imbalanced hormones, or traumatic experiences.

Whatever the cause, experts agree that the brains of bipolar individuals are wired differently. Individuals with bipolar disorder have a biological abnormality in the function and structure of certain brain circuits. The brain is made up of billions of nerve cells (neurons) that move a constant stream of information from one to another. Chemical messengers in the brain, known as neurotransmitters, transmit signals between neurons. Neurotransmitters play a crucial role in emotional health, are involved in brain functions, and also help in the functioning of the human body. The abnormal brain circuits identified in bipolar brains cause certain neurotransmitters in the brain to be dysfunctional.

Neurotransmitters

Scientists have identified serotonin, dopamine, and norepinephrine as the three prevalent neurotransmitters involved in mood regulation, stress responses, pleasure, reward, and cognitive functions like concentration, attention, and executive functions. When the levels or density of these neurotransmitters are not "normal," the result is the manifestation of bipolar disorder.

Serotonin is a brain chemical that is connected to several body functions such as wakefulness, sleep, sexual activity, eating, learning, impulsivity, and memory. Any abnormal rise or fall in the serotonin levels of a human brain can lead to mood disorders, which can elevate medical conditions like depression and bipolar disorder.

Dopamine has consistently been linked with the part of the brain that controls the human pleasure center. This neurotransmitter helps control body movements and patterns of thought, and it also regulates how hormones are released. Abnormal dopamine activity in your brain may explain the symptoms of bipolar disorder.

Norepinephrine plays a role in cognition, mood, emotions, movement, and blood pressure. Imbalance in norepinephrine causes difficulty concentrating, fatigue, anxiety, apathy, and depression.

Research on Bipolar Disorder

Positron emission tomography (PET) is a brain-imaging technique that has been used to measure the monoamine density of cells that release the brain chemicals dopamine, serotonin, and norepinephrine. "By performing PET scans in areas of the brain in which monoamine-releasing cells are concentrated, an approximate 30 percent increase in density of these cells was found in the brains of bipolar people even when not having symptoms" (Evidence of Brain Chemistry Abnormalities 2005).

The altered brain chemistry due to the excess monoamine cells directly affects cognitive and social functions. Studies continue to determine which kinds of monoamine cells are involved that produce serotonin and norepinephrine. Those findings could help define specific subtypes of bipolar disorder and aid in the development of medications and drug combinations that target a specific patient's personal brain chemistry to alleviate symptoms.

Magnetic resonance imaging (MRI) technology has been used to view the brains of individuals with bipolar disorder. The results of these studies showed gray-matter abnormalities in various regions of the brain. Gray matter is a major component of the central nervous system, consisting of neuronal cell bodies. "Scientists have found gray matter deficits in the ventromedial prefrontal regions of the bipolar brain (located in the rear of the front part of the brain, inside the cortex and atop the orbits of the eyes), and in the anterior limbic cortices of the brain" (Narita 2011).

The particular brain areas affected with gray-matter deficits each affect certain brain functions. The ventromedial prefrontal regions of the brain affect concentration, inhibition, emotions, behavior, and learning, and the anterior limbic cortices affect smell, agitation, emotional control, and memory. By studying the gray matter found in the brains of bipolar and non-bipolar individuals, scientists hope to correlate the volume of gray matter with the duration of bipolar illness and the number of episodes.

Genetic Predisposition

Bipolar disorder has a strong but as-of-yet-unknown tie to DNA. There is an overwhelming amount of evidence that bipolar disorder can be inherited or "runs in the family." "The evidence for a genetic predisposition to bipolar disorder is so strong that based on studies of twins, an estimated 80 percent of the risk is inherited. If one of your parents or siblings has the disorder, your chances of having it are four to ten times greater than they would be if no one in your family had it" (Haycock 2010, 60). The author concludes that approximately 33 percent of children who have a parent with bipolar disorder will get it.

Gary comments about the possibility that his kids may have inherited bipolar disorder.

What? Are you kidding me? Having to deal with my bipolar disorder is hard enough without worrying my kids may have it also. I have talked to each of my kids about bipolar disorder. They have seen me battling bipolar disorder, visited me in the hospital, seen me manic and depressed. I pray to whatever power there is in the universe that none of my children are bipolar!

Scientists are trying to find genes that are involved in causing bipolar disorder in hopes of finding genetic markers that will help people know their risk of developing the disorder. A combination of both genetic research and neuroimaging studies are being pursued to help define both the genetic components of this illness and their relationship with specific brain chemical markers that define a "chemical fingerprint" for bipolar patients.

The important thing to remember is this—what's inherited in bipolar disorder is not the illness itself but vulnerability. And whether the person does or does not get the illness depends on what's happening in that person's life. Interventions, like medications or family interventions that reduce stress and introduce structure in the life of a person who is vulnerable to bipolar illness, could be very helpful and may prevent or delay the onset of the illness.

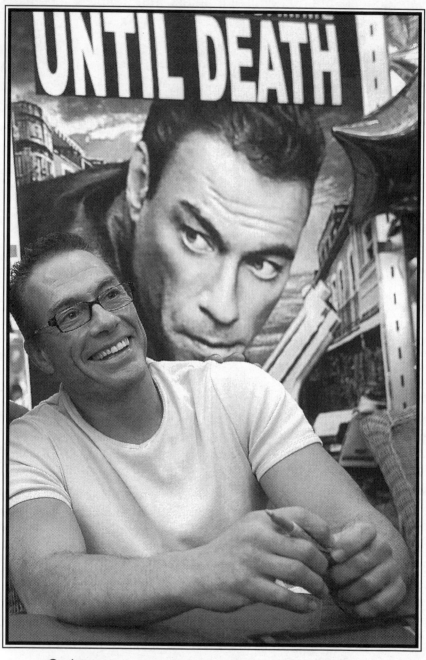

God gave me a great body, and it's my duty to take care of my physical temple.
—Jean-Claude Van Damme, actor

CHAPTER 7

Train Your Body

Consistent application of several or all of the following actions will tune your body and improve your physical health. Your mind and body are a unit; exercising your body improves your mood and benefits your mind. Prepare yourself for the battles ahead. Every morning when you wake up, remind yourself to adopt the mind-set of a warrior and act accordingly. You may find it easier to accomplish these actions if you put them in your schedule on a consistent basis—for example, take walks at lunch and get fresh air at the same time.

Exercise Several Days a Week

If you take care of your body, it will take care of you. Take walks, run, ride your bike, lift weights, dance, use the elliptical, do yoga, play basketball—do anything you enjoy that gets the blood pumping.

Get Fresh Air

Getting fresh air every day clears your head, calms you down, and helps you appreciate the fact that you are alive on this awesome earth.

Stretch Several Times a Day

Stretch your arms, legs, torso, and neck several times a day. This is especially important after sitting for extended periods of time.

Build the Core

The core is one of the most important parts of the body to exercise and strengthen. In anatomy, the *core* refers to the body except for the legs and arms. Functional movements are highly dependent on the core, and lack of core development can result in a predisposition to injury. The major muscles of the core reside in the area of the belly, the mid—and lower back (not the shoulders), and peripherally the hips, the shoulders, and the neck.

We are all different physically, and our energy levels vary from person to person. Start at whatever level you are now, and slowly increase your prowess. Build a strong core. Work the stomach muscles. Something as simple as sucking in the stomach and then pushing it out while standing in line or driving helps. It takes a while, but it is worth it. Besides the physical benefits, a strong core increases your willpower and sharpens your gut instincts.

Use Alcohol and Drugs Intelligently

Approximately 40 percent of us who are bipolar abuse alcohol or drugs, many of us doing so to self-medicate. However, hangovers suck, and being high much of the time distorts your reality.

It is not necessary to stop drinking or doing drugs completely. The key is to not indulge and drink too much alcohol or smoke too much pot, or whatever. Stop overdoing alcohol or drugs and live by the saying, "I went from too much to not too much."

What you do to exercise your mind and your body is important, but what you *don't* do to your mind and body is more important. By avoiding anything that is harmful to your body and your mind, you will not obstruct the way your body naturally functions, and in return, your body will take care of you.

As an alternative to self-medicating with drugs and alcohol, learn to use bipolar medications to your advantage instead. Bipolar medications are very powerful pharmaceutical drugs, and if used intelligently, they can give you a very good, legal buzz. Consider the medicine as a blessing instead of a curse.

Make Love

Having sex with someone I like and who likes me back always makes me feel better. How about you? Physical closeness as well as pleasure is good for us, and don't forget the dopamine released during sex. It is a natural "high" that is your body's way of saying, "Thanks. I needed that!"

Take Vitamins

There are definite benefits in taking vitamins. Vitamin B aids in cell metabolism and harvests energy to create and support your body's chemical reactions. A lot of people are deficient in Vitamin D due to a lack of sunlight, and Vitamin D helps with the immune system. Vitamin C protects against immune system deficiencies, cardiovascular disease, prenatal health problems, and eye disease.

Drink Water

It is important to flush your system and hydrate. Cut back on drinking soft drinks and drink more water. Water is very helpful when you are trying to lose weight because it reduces your hunger. It also helps your mind function more effectively.

Eat Healthily

It is not necessary to give up pizza or anything you love to eat or drink. Eat protein (steak, chicken, eggs, cheese), as well as salads, veggies, and fruit. Cut back on the carbohydrates (white bread, pasta, sweets). Balance is the key.

Get Your Thyroid Checked

Thyroid disease is associated with bipolar disorder and can actually cause bipolar disorder as well as diabetes. Anyone who is bipolar should get his or her thyroid checked for a hypothyroid (slow) or hyperthyroid (fast). There is a simple blood test that measures the amount of thyroid-stimulating hormone (TSH) in the body. Thyroid medicine will correct either a hypo—or hyperthyroid condition, both of which can mimic the symptoms of bipolar disorder.

One excellent benefit of treating a hypothyroid condition is that it speeds up the metabolism and helps with weight loss. Make an appointment with an endocrinologist and get your thyroid checked out.

Natural Herbs and Spices

Fish Oil and Omega-3 Fatty Acids: Fish oil is proven to have positive effects on depression. Food sources of omega-3 fatty acids include salmon, albacore tuna, flaxseed and walnuts.

Garlic: Use garlic as a cure-all for whatever ails you. Garlic cures colds, coughs, aches and pains, and infections. Garlic wards off heart disease, improves cholesterol, and lowers blood pressure. Bulk up on the garlic when you start to feel sick. One tasty way to eat garlic is to cut up fresh garlic, cook it in the oven with olive oil until slightly crispy, and put butter on it.

Cinnamon: Cinnamon lowers blood sugar, detoxifies the system, and stimulates brain function.

Curry: This spice helps with joint health, acts as an anti-inflammatory, antioxidant, and anti-tumor remedy.

Cardamom: Increased circulation and improved energy are two benefits of cardamom. It is also considered an aphrodisiac in the Middle East.

Cloves: Cloves improve digestion and alleviate toothaches, sore throats, diarrhea, and stomach cramps.

Take Showers or Baths

It is surprising how good it feels to take a shower or bath. Cleansing yourself with water relaxes you and makes you feel clean and refreshed. Take a shower or bath and feel better every time. Just splashing cold water on your face is reviving.

Brush Your Teeth and Use Mouthwash

Fresh, minty breath is good for warding off disease and tooth decay and makes you feel better about yourself.

Shed Extra Pounds

Your body functions better and your energy levels are put to better use when you are not overweight. Most diets are predicated on minimizing the number of calories that you take in. A diet that consistently works and does not require starving yourself is to eat only fresh fruits and vegetables for two weeks. Five people I know, myself included, lost at least ten pounds on this diet. It is important to eat several times a day when on this diet, which kicks your metabolism into gear. The diet is actually very healthy. Two weeks is not that long of a time, if you think about it. For any type of diet you attempt, drink a lot of water because it reduces your hunger and helps cleanse your system.

As mentioned in the "Bipolar Disorder Facts and Statistics" section in chapter 6, approximately 25 percent of people with bipolar disorder are grossly fat or overweight (obese). Also, people with bipolar disorder are approximately three times more likely to develop diabetes than are members of the general population. The good news is that both obesity and diabetes can be controlled. By changing your diet, you can effectively lose weight and fight diabetes.

Animal Lovers

Caring for an animal can provide companionship and be therapeutic and rewarding. It is nice to have a feeling of being loved every time you come home. Unconditional love from a pal who needs you and always cares can be a key to maintaining consistent mental health.

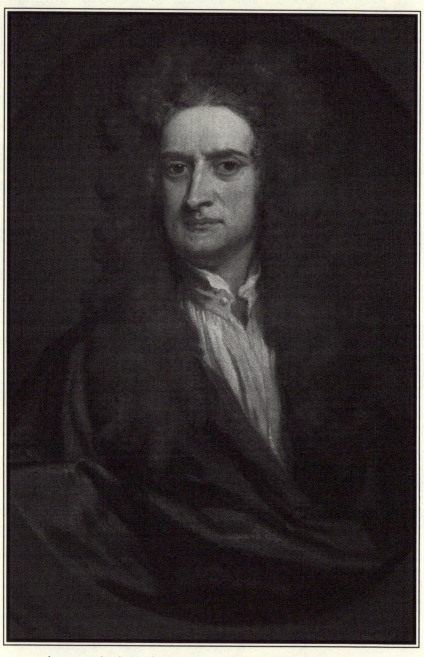

I can calculate the motion of heavenly bodies, but not the madness of people.
—Isaac Newton, mathematician, physicist

CHAPTER 8
Train Your Mind

Your mind is your most powerful weapon. Your thoughts are the only thing over which you can exert complete control. Whatever you think and believe becomes a reality and rules your life. For those of us who are bipolar, however, it is a paradox that we must use our minds to fight a disease that at times has the power to take control of them.

> *Happiness is an attitude. We either make ourselves miserable, or happy and strong. The amount of work is the same.*
>
> —Francesca Reigler

The intent of this chapter is to present a number of strategies and techniques that can be used to improve your emotional well-being, decrease stress, and bring you happiness and joy. These strategies and techniques were gathered from self-help books written by best-selling authors such as Napoleon Hill, Miguel Ruiz, Carlos Castaneda, and others.

The Path with Heart

> Anything is one of a million paths. Therefore, a warrior must always keep in mind that a path is only a path; if he feels that he should not follow it, he must not stay with it under any conditions. His decision to keep on that path or to leave it must be free of fear or ambition. He must look at every path closely and deliberately. There is a question that a warrior has to ask, mandatorily. Does this path have a heart?
>
> All paths are the same: they lead nowhere. However a path without a heart is never enjoyable. On the other hand, a path with heart is easy—it does not make a warrior work at liking it; it makes for a joyful journey; as long as a man follows it, he is one with it. (Castaneda 1998, 19)

With regard to making decisions in our lives as to what paths to follow and what paths to avoid, the above words of Carlos Castaneda ring true and cannot be refuted. Use your heart as a GPS to guide you in the direction of your dreams. You will know when you are achieving the results you are striving for when your heart leaps for joy. A path with heart is formed by deliberately selecting a number of things that you want to involve yourself with: relationships, vocations, hobbies, arts, anything that really connects your heart with the world. The criteria for selection are peace, joy, and strength.

> *It is only with the heart that one can see rightly; what is essential is invisible to the eye.*
> —Antoine de Saint-Exupery

Death Is Stalking You

Time waits for no man.
—Abraham Lincoln

A warrior uses death as her most important advisor. She routinely asks the following questions:

- If all I have is this moment, how do I want to use it?
- Is this the best I can do?
- Is this activity worthy of my life?
- If I died right now, would my death respect me?

In a world where death is the hunter, there is no time for regrets or doubts. There is only time for decisions. Our most costly mistake as average men is indulging in a sense of immortality. It is as though we believe that if we don't think about death we can protect ourselves from it. Only the idea of death makes a warrior sufficiently detached so that he is capable of abandoning himself to anything. He knows his death is stalking him and won't give him time to cling to anything so he tries without craving all of everything. (Teachings n.d.)

Using death as an advisor helps you to focus on what matters most, to make things clear. Other concerns pale in comparison. Meaning wells up from the heart, and you clearly understand how you want to live.

The following words from the movie *Walk the Line* about the life of Johnny Cash "brings home" the importance of using death as an advisor:

All right, let's bring it home. If you was hit by a truck, and you were lying out in that gutter dying, and you had time to sing one song, one song people would remember before you're dirt, one song that would let God know what you felt about your time here on earth, one song that would sum you up, are you telling me that's the song you'd sing, that same Jimmy Davis tune we hear on the radio all day, about your peace within and how it's real and how you're gonna shout it? Or, would you sing something different, something real, something you felt? 'Cause I'm telling you right now that's the kind of song people want to hear. That's the kind of song that truly saves people. It ain't got nothing to do with believing in God, Mr. Cash. It has to do with believing in yourself.

As I write this section in a Starbucks, a spry-looking lady of about sixty barely escaped slipping on the wet concrete outside and having a nasty fall and perhaps splitting her skull. Luckily, she caught herself. Death is always a stone throw's away. Our time on earth is limited, and there is no time to be mediocre. Embrace your own essence and grab life by the horns!

Always Do Your Best

I do the very best I know how, the very best I can, and I mean to keep doing so until the end.
—Abraham Lincoln

Doing your best in everything you do is a habit you can groom—the more you practice, the better you get. By consistently doing your best, your life improves dramatically, your self-respect increases, and so does your productivity. Doing your best is about taking action and doing what you love to do because it's the action that makes you happy.

> Always do your best. For sure, you can always do your best. And your best changes all the time—when you are sick or tired, your best is different than when you are awake and fresh. But by always doing your best, you are going to be content with yourself. If you make the choice to do your best and believe it, that is your best. You have the power to make the choice. And magic begins to happen in your life. This is the mastery of life. This is the path to personal freedom.
>
> Under any circumstance simply do your best and you will avoid self-judgment, self-abuse and regret. Everything you have ever learned you have learned by repetition. You learned to write, to drive, and even to walk by repetition. Practice makes the master. By doing your best you become the master. If you do your best always, over and over again, you will become a master of transformation. (Ruiz 1997, 76)

I can tell when I do my best. I feel a sense of accomplishment. I am able to unclutter my mind and redirect my energy into the next logical step or task that I should take to accomplish my goals.

Do your best every day, accept that you have done what you could, and be proud of yourself for your efforts. Even when you haven't done your best, forgive yourself, move on, and commit to trying harder next time. Make doing your best a challenge in your daily life. If you approach a task, even something as minute as tying your shoes, with the mind-set that you are going to do it right the first time, it will keep you from spending the time redoing it. As the saying goes. "Time is money." If you do your best over and over again, you will enrich your life, be more productive, and improve your self-esteem.

Self-Importance Is Your Greatest Enemy

Self-importance is the belief that you are more important than everyone else. Exaggerating one's importance is often accompanied by arrogance, conceit, and egotistical behavior. Cockiness is for fools. If you think about it, our self-importance causes us to be offended by other people, what they say, and what they do. This is a huge waste of energy and our precious time. It makes us weak.

Self-importance causes us to do the following:

- feel offended
- defend our image
- complain
- reject ourselves
- suffer needlessly
- feel sorry for ourselves (self-pity)
- think negatively
- make everyone else wrong
- defend our opinions
- gossip about ourselves and others

How much time do we spend complaining about our problems, feeling offended about something someone said or did, or feeling sad and playing "Poor Me"?

For example, you spend all day thinking about a girlfriend or boyfriend who pissed you off, whether you should stay with him or her, and wondering if you are wasting your time with this person. That night, you get into a car accident, and the last thought you have before you die is, *Man, I wasted the whole day feeling lousy when I should have been having fun, enjoying myself, and being thankful for just being here.*

Reducing self-importance frees up energy that you can rechannel into furthering your goals, reduces negative thought patterns, eliminates needless anger and suffering, and increases happiness. To free mental and emotional energy, annihilate the self-important patterns of behavior such as the presentation and defense of the self in everyday life, excessive routines, the tremendous insistence on the concerns of the self, and the incessant preoccupation with romantic courtship.

Following are four techniques for reducing self-importance.

Shush the internal dialogue

Internal dialogue is the incessant voice running through our heads that has been programmed and groomed to focus on our egos ever since we started to think. Our minds constantly focus on our internal dialogue (self-talk). Our self-talk programs and shapes our self-concept. For example, if you believe you are worthy and strong, you will live up to that truth. On the other hand, if you criticize yourself and tell yourself you will never get what you want, you won't.

Stop defending your self-image

Over the years you have built an idealized self-image that you defend as "me." In this image are packed all the things you want to see as true about yourself; banished from it are all the shameful, guilty, and fear-provoking aspects that threaten your self-confidence. Much time is spent in self-help, trying to turn a bad self-image into a good one. As reasonable as that sounds, all self-images have the same pitfall: they keep reminding you of who you were, not who you are. The whole idea of *I, me*, and *mine* was erected on memories, and these memories are not really you.

Stop having to be right or wrong

To reduce self-importance, stop trying to make yourself right and others wrong. Everyone is a product of his or her environment and has formed an opinion about almost everything. If you quit caring whether you are right or wrong, then you will stop judging yourself and others and trying to prove that your opinion is superior to theirs.

Accept the way you are

We are our own worst enemies because of the habit we have of criticizing and judging ourselves. We criticize ourselves hundreds of times a day without even realizing it. Our critic keeps us in line. Think about it—how often do you give yourself a hard time over past events, things you said, or past actions? The more emotion that was invested in the event, the more we criticize ourselves for the same transgression over and over again. Reduce the amount of time you spend criticizing yourself, and your mind will be more at peace.

Stalk Yourself

The "Art of Stalking" is a set of procedures and attitudes that enables you to get the best of any conceivable situation. For this discussion, stalking results in positive results and is not associated with doing any kind of harm to other people.

John explains stalking to his son.

> My twenty-year-old son and I were sitting in a booth at Denny's waiting for his girlfriend to show up. He was getting irate because she was late. We reminisced, as we always did when the subject of being late came up, about his mom (my ex), who was habitually late and drove me and the kids crazy. He kept looking at his watch, and I knew he was going to jump his girlfriend's case when she arrived.
>
> He calmed down a little bit when I asked him when he had to leave and go to work. He said he had an hour before he had to leave, so there was no big hurry. I asked him if he had ever heard about stalking someone, not in the sense of intending to do them harm or being a predator, but in terms of gaining energy and not wasting it. He said, "No, what do you mean?" I explained that stalking is a set of procedures and attitudes that would enable him to get the best of any situation.
>
> I told him an example of stalking would be not to act irritated at his girlfriend when she arrived—don't show any negative emotion at all, but convince her it doesn't bother you one bit that she is late. If

> she says she is sorry for being late, simply say, "No problem. My dad and I were just talking. I don't have to leave for work for a while." I explained to him that acting in this manner, even if he was irritated on the inside, would keep him from wasting his energy being negative, she wouldn't feel bad, and we would have a much better time eating breakfast together. By following this course of action he would have successfully stalked her because she would treat him better and be more understanding when he did something that pissed her off.
>
> Then I drove home the most important benefit of stalking. I told him that by stalking his girlfriend, he was actually stalking himself. By using his mind in a disciplined manner and choosing not to take her arriving late personally, he wouldn't cause himself or anyone else at the table needless suffering.

Strange to stalk yourself, isn't it? Try it and see how effective it can be.

> Because your mind is especially subject to the dominating influences in your environment, you must take control over those influences by developing beneficial mental habits. The process of controlling your habits is miraculous. It translates the power of thought into action. But if your habits are poor or bad, they can bring misery and failure. Your success depends on the strength and quality of your controlled habits. (Hill 1983, 133)

Erase Personal History

For most people, personal history must be constantly renewed by telling parents, relatives, friends, and coworkers everything that we do or that happens to us. As a result, they pin us down with their thoughts and expectations. Erasing personal history frees us from the encumbering thoughts of other people. We are not defined by our past—the future is what matters!

Start keeping personal things to yourself that you normally would have shared with someone else. Slowly over time, tell people less and less about what you do and who you are. In this manner, you can begin to erase your personal history. Camouflage your personal history to keep from being pinned down by other people's thoughts or expectations. You need not be pigeonholed because you are bipolar, for example.

The benefits of erasing your personal history include:

- No one pins you down with his or her thoughts or expectations.
- You can re-create yourself into whomever you want to be.
- Forgetting the past allows you to focus on what is happening now and stop wasting your energy mulling over past events.

Explanations are a sign of weakness. With every explanation, there is a hidden apology. Don't gossip about yourself or about others. They don't need to know everything. Much of it is none of their business. An average man believes that his explanations of life will enable him to survive, but explanations are a meaningless waste of time.

Understanding is a matter of experience, not the result of explanations. By erasing personal history, no explanations are needed, and nobody is angry or disillusioned with our acts.

Note that an exception to keeping things to yourself is if you want to talk to others like friends or family and gain their thoughts and insights about a particular situation.

Autosuggestion

In his best-selling book *Think and Grow Rich*, Napoleon Hill explains a process called autosuggestion, which relies on the principle, "What you focus on, you attract."

> Autosuggestion is the process of voluntarily fixing your attention upon a definite major purpose of a positive nature and forcing your mind through daily habits of thought, to dwell on that subject. (Hill 1983, p.143)

The dominating thoughts that you hold in your conscious mind act to magnetize your subconscious, and these "magnets" attract the forces, people, and circumstances of life that you desire. This is why visualizations, affirmations, and repeated images can have such a powerful effect in your life.

The "language" of the subconscious mind is feelings and emotions. Emotions are either positive or negative; both cannot occupy the mind at the same time. By focusing on positive emotions and banishing negative ones, you save up energy to expend on your definite major purpose instead of wasting your energy on negativity. There are seven positive and seven negative emotions that your subconscious understands.

Positive Emotions
desire
faith
love
sex
enthusiasm
romance
hope

Negative Emotions
fear
jealousy
hatred
greed
vengefulness
superstition
anger

The process of autosuggestion consists of the following steps:

1. Decide on a major purpose you want to accomplish. Choose something you really want!

2. Say this affirmation out loud: "My subconscious mind is my partner in success."

3. Concentrate on your major purpose and visualize what it will look and feel like when it comes true.

4. Flood your mind with positive emotions.

5. Be alert and receptive of the ideas, people, and circumstances that show up in your life to aid you in the achievement of your major purpose.

6. Take action.

7. Spend ten minutes every day for a month following these steps.

Face Fear Head On

Courage is being scared to death, but saddling up anyway.
—John Wayne

Anytime you come up on something and the only thing that keeps you from doing it is fear, your decision is automatically made. You look it straight in the eye and proceed in that direction.

Too often we allow fear, worry, and doubts to dominate and define our lives. We allow them to steal our joy, our sleep, and our precious dreams. There are several steps you can take to face fear.

- Get comfortable with fear.
- Make your dominant thoughts positive.
- Don't give attention, energy or time to fear.
- Don't dwell on scarcity.
- Laugh at your fear.
- Tell yourself that in one hundred years, whatever happens as a result of your facing your fear won't matter.
- View life as a wild adventure.
- Plan to be great.

> Your emotional posture is a major influence regarding how others relate to you and how you experience the world. If you're afraid of doing something, you're likely to avoid it or be timid doing it. At the same time, if you don't acknowledge negative feelings, you allow them to fester and thus diminish physical, mental, and emotional health. Worry, for example, warps energy. Enmeshed in the furrows of worry, people constantly struggle with, and tear apart, stabilizing energies such as control, patience, and timing. Thus people become accessible and lose their balance and their wits. (Feather 2006, 234)

Taking action in spite of your fears is extremely difficult. A powerful technique that can help you face your fear is to visualize a positive end result and practicing until you know exactly what you need to do to succeed. For example, many of us are afraid of public speaking. In order to face that fear, practice, practice, and practice some more in front of a mirror. Plan your speech in your mind. When you prepare your speech, say something funny in the beginning. The audience will relax, and so will you. A couple of other tips are when you first walk up to the podium or in front of your audience, take three breaths before you begin to speak. Also, instead of standing still and not moving while delivering your speech, say a paragraph and then move to the left or to the right a few steps and then continue. Visualize the speech going great.

Many actors and actresses use beta-blockers when they perform. These are pills that slow down the heart rate. I took a beta-blocker when I gave a speech for my dad's funeral in front of over fifty people. Of course, I also followed all the advice from the previous paragraph, and the end result was that I nailed the speech. Your psychiatrist can prescribe beta-blockers if you are so inclined.

Running the Bipolar Marathon

Battling bipolar disorder is a lifelong fight that can be compared to running a marathon. Marathon runners train, train, train, and then run the race to the best of their ability. Follow the advice below for running your personal bipolar marathon.

1. There are good days and bad days, and sometimes you can't tell the difference until you start.

2. Contrary to popular belief, sleep is not overrated—not in the slightest.

3. Don't forget to breathe.

4. Just because it's raining doesn't mean you should cry.

5. Nobody ever said it was easy.

6. Pain is temporary, but pride lasts a lifetime—sometimes even two.

7. Create a plan and stick to it. It may not always work, but if you stay focused and relaxed, it will end up just fine.

8. You've got to try no matter what happens. In the end, you'll have bigger regrets from not trying at all.

9. Strength and courage blossom from the seeds of adversity.

10. Sometimes it's the little things that make the big differences.

11. Getting to the starting line is usually a lot harder than getting to the finish.

12. Listen to your body and listen to your mind. And make sure you know when they are lying to you.

13. You can't change the past, and you won't alter the future. Enjoy right now right now and always be positive!

14. Smile—it is contagious and increases endorphins. It actually takes more muscles and energy to frown.

15. It is okay to cry.

16. Don't forget to eat, especially breakfast. Food can dictate your mood.

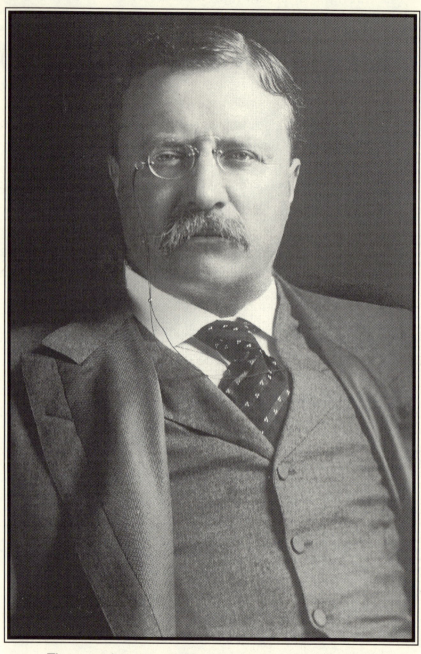

The most important single ingredient in the formula of success is knowing how to get along with people.
—Theodore Roosevelt, rough rider, president

CHAPTER 9
Teamwork

Teaming up with your support personnel, like your significant other, family members, and friends, can be a powerful weapon in your war against bipolar illness. It also carries great risk. Admitting to others that you need help and, more important, that they are part of your contingency plan takes great trust, both in yourself and in them. It is essential, though. This is a great leap into the unknown for you and them, so pick your team carefully, accepting that this is a lifelong condition and that there will be times when you need them.

Again, You Aren't Alone

How does bipolar disorder affect the people closest to you?

The people closest to you are the ones who are most affected by your bipolar disorder. They take the brunt of your actions and live with the consequences. Understanding and untangling the complex array of issues and the emotions that surround them is difficult and usually takes much time and effort. For your loved ones, the issue often comes down to finding ways to maintain a loving relationship through the long process of finding effective treatment and achieving greater stability.

Consider the havoc that your bipolar illness can rain upon the people closest to you.

- They have to deal with your impaired judgment during a manic phase of the bipolar cycle. Impaired judgment is exhibited through such conduct as impulsive spending and acting out sexually.
- You may be unable to maintain gainful employment. Significant others or family members sometimes end up dealing with that financial burden.
- You may direct anger at them due to your imbalance, uncertainty, and inability to function. Anger can take the form of verbal abuse and instantaneous rage.
- You may physically abuse the people closest to you. Physical abuse is more common if you are not properly medicated and are utilizing mind-altering substances.

While the behaviors that lead to the bipolar diagnosis vary widely in severity, they are sometimes very disturbing, frightening, threatening, or annoying. Sometimes sustaining the relationship is complicated by financial insecurity, infidelity, alcoholism, addiction, abusiveness, criminal activity, and other factors that may be associated with the illness.

Being bipolar can wreck your life and the lives of the ones closest to you. Teaming up with them and working together to combat the enemy can keep your relationships intact, keep you and them safe, speed up your recovery, and minimize the negative effects of the disease. Working together is as important to you as it is to them; it makes good sense to include them in your treatment plan. They want you to get better because they love you. They also want to protect themselves. This chapter presents a number of ways to involve your loved ones in helping you manage your disease.

It is important to remember that, in some circumstances, trying to work together with the person or people closest to you is not a good move. Perhaps your relationships with them are exasperating your condition due to the stresses caused by a bad relationship and creating more triggers for your mood swings. If you know in your gut that working with them is more detrimental than helpful and that you are not making your decision just because of bipolar symptoms, distance yourself from them and revise your treatment (battle) plan accordingly. You can always renew your relationship once you are back in control of your faculties.

How Can the People Closest to You Help You Manage Your Illness?

Be on your side

The most important thing the people closest to you can do is to be on your side. Trust is paramount for teamwork. If they offer love, support, understanding, and tolerance, they will gain your trust, and you can team up and battle bipolar disorder together. By assuring you that you are not alone, you will not be as stressed and will have a better chance to win the battles against the enemy.

Alternatively, if they convey that they are holier than you or nag, preach, and lecture, most likely you will take just so much and shut out the rest.

Be part of your contingency plan

As mentioned in chapter 3, the first and most important action to take if you are bipolar is to create a contingency plan. Recruiting the person or people you trust the most to come to your aid in the event of a bipolar episode is common sense. A benefit of enlisting the help of the person who is around you most often is that he or she is more apt to detect symptoms and bring them to your attention. The ones who know you the best may be able to help you put your contingency plan into effect and stop dangerous symptoms like thoughts of suicide, spending sprees, violence, and promiscuity from happening.

Become knowledgeable of the disease

The more knowledge that the people closest to you have of bipolar disorder, the better they will be able to assist you in fighting the war. You are their best resource. The best place to start is to talk with them about your symptoms and describe how bipolar disorder manifests itself in your life. Talk to them about your past episodes and what you were thinking about and feeling as you became manic or depressed.

Finding a bipolar support group in your city and going to meetings together is an excellent resource for learning about the disease. Also, reading books and doing research on the Internet can teach about bipolar disorder and provide invaluable resources.

Use the bipolar battle plan outlined in this book

By using the bipolar battle plan outlined in this book and working as a team to fight the war against bipolar disorder, you can prevent yourself from having episodes and help yourself (and the people helping you) achieve your dreams.

Understand that it takes time to recover from an episode

Neither you nor your loved ones should expect an immediate, 100 percent recovery after an episode. In any illness, there is a period of convalescence. There may be relapses and times of tension and resentment. It takes time and fortitude to recover from an episode. Many times, a huge factor is medication. If the episode was severe, then you may have been heavily medicated with high dosages of strong pharmaceutical medications to bring your symptoms into check. When you become stable, your doctor will reduce these large dosages or discontinue this powerful medicine and reinstitute maintenance dosages of another medication. Weaning yourself from high dosages of any medicine is difficult, sometimes extremely so.

John talks about returning home from the psychiatric hospital after an episode:

> I had a manic episode that resulted in me being involuntarily admitted to a psychiatric hospital. They dosed me with some powerful medicines and, four days later, when I stabilized I was discharged. After I got home, I had to deal with side effects from the medications. My hands were trembling so much I couldn't sign my name on checks and withdrawal slips. I was taking a class for college and I could only

concentrate for a short amount of time. Not to mention returning to work. It took me a couple of weeks to start feeling myself again.

Help you watch for symptoms

Make a pact with your significant other or person you will be around the most that if you begin exhibiting manic or depressive symptoms, they should bring it to your attention. Make sure they have a copy of your contingency plan and are clear about what they should do if you spiral out of control.

Support your bipolar recovery plan

Your support team needs to offer love, support, and understanding in the recovery plan, regardless of the method chosen. For example, some people choose to take meds; some choose not to. Each has advantages and disadvantages (more side effects versus higher instances of relapse, for example). Expressing disapproval of the method chosen will only deepen your feeling that anything you do will be wrong.

Urge you to stop (or reduce) drinking alcohol or taking drugs

Alcohol and drugs can be the most likely contributors to your bipolar symptoms. Reducing how much you are drinking or using drugs is an intelligent approach to slowing down your episode. However, sometimes you may use them to self-medicate. Your support person can help you by urging you to stop or at least slow down your alcohol or drug consumption. Note that they should not try to take it away from you or try to hide it. Usually, this will push you into a state of desperation or depression. In the end, you will find new ways of getting more drugs or alcohol if you want them badly enough. On the other hand, if excessive use of drugs or alcohol is really a problem, they should not let you persuade them to use drugs or drink with you on the grounds that it will make you use less. It rarely does. When they condone the use of drugs or alcohol, it is likely to cause you to put off seeking necessary help.

Get support for themselves

One significant other says, "On the up days, I couldn't ask for a better partner. On the down days, I just keep telling myself he has a disease [and] I need to be here for him."

If you are a support person, it's important that you take some steps to support yourself as well.

- You may dearly miss the person you fell in love with. Keep in mind that with proper treatments and your support, that person will come back to you.
- Find your own therapist to help guide you through the hard times.
- Look for a support group for partners of bipolar sufferers.
- Go with your spouse to a few of his or her therapy sessions and talk to the therapist. Ask questions and listen to the therapist's conclusions or views of your spouse's care.
- Find time for yourself with such things as hobbies, walks, jogging, sports, and writing, and vent a bit of frustrated energy.

- When your partner is in a healthy mental state, talk to him or her about your needs and hurts. Don't be confrontational and don't blame, but tell him or her how you feel about things from your perspective.

Convince you that you are bipolar

If you reach the stage where you are convinced that you are bipolar, then the battle is halfway won. Once you are convinced that you are bipolar, which usually takes a disastrous episode or two, then you will be much more willing to take medication as well as seek other treatments. Therefore, if you are in denial, your loved ones should do what they can to convince you. However, they should not use the "If you love me . . ." appeal. Saying that you should do what they want you to do is like saying, "If you loved me, you would not have diabetes."

Guard against taking the "Holier than thou" attitude

Don't take the "I am better than you" attitude. Because of your bipolar condition, you are likely to have an emotional sensitivity such that you judge other people's attitudes toward you more by actions, even small ones, than by spoken words.

Not try to make you dependent on them

Your loved ones should not try to protect you from situations that may be stressful or depressing. One of the quickest ways they can push you away is to make you feel like they want you to be dependent on them.

Let you decide for yourself how to handle situations

You must learn for yourself what works best for you, especially in social situations. Your loved ones should let you decide for yourself whether to answer questions or to gracefully say, "I'd prefer to discuss something else." Your loved ones' role here would be to have an upfront discussion with you about what you might have to face.

Respect your independence

Your loved ones should not do for you what you can do for yourself. They cannot take the medicine for you; they cannot feel your feelings for you; they can't solve your problems for you. They shouldn't try. They should not remove problems before you can face them, solve them, or suffer the consequences. This is your life. They are on your team, but this is your battle to fight.

Sometimes the stresses are too great, and separation or divorce must be considered. This is a very important decision. Talk to your psychiatrist and trusted friends before making the decision. Try separation first, and wait to see how you feel several months later before getting divorced. If you have children, you need to be a good father or mother and keep their well-being in mind. Also, many times there are financial ramifications.

Arm Your Team with Your Contingency Plan

No plan is useful unless it is enacted. In the back of this book is your personal contingency plan. Create it with your team's involvement, make them understand how important it is, and, critically, *make copies*! If they don't have this plan handy, they will be shooting in the dark. This is important information that they need at their disposal—your psychiatrist's phone number, other contacts, medications, and so on. Have it at the ready and in the hands of those you most trust.

CHAPTER 10
Psychiatric Hospitals

Knowledge about the ins and outs of psychiatric hospitals is an important weapon in your bipolar battle plan. Bipolar episodes sometimes end with a stay in the psychiatric hospital, either by voluntarily checking in or being involuntarily committed. Hopefully you will never need to go into the hospital. However, if you do, knowing what to expect is very helpful and can speed up your recovery.

It is an extremely tough decision to check into a psychiatric hospital. However, when bipolar symptoms become severe and you are in the throes of a full-blown manic or depressive episode, checking yourself in may be the smartest move you can make. Being in a psychiatric hospital is similar to being in any other hospital: you are there to heal, calm down, and be safe.

If you think you should check into a psychiatric hospital, do it. If you feel you do not have the strength to do it alone, find someone who supports you to take you there.

Get help so that you can live to fight another day. Dire consequences of not getting help can include attempted suicide, self-mutilation, physical violence, or other unbelievably catastrophic results. Recall that 30 percent of us who are bipolar attempt suicide.

Advice from Fellow Bipolars

Four bipolar individuals who have been in a psychiatric hospital talk about their experiences and offer advice.

Gary

I was out of control, belligerent, and having hallucinations about being on a mission from God. I got in a fight in a bar with a bouncer who was giving me shit, and the cops came. I told them the bouncer was the devil. The police took me to a psychiatric hospital where I was involuntarily admitted against my will. It took four days but, after I was medicated and under control, I told the doctor I had to get back to work and he signed my discharge papers. The nurses and staff were very good to me, smiling and telling me to take it easy and things would improve. I'm not sure what would have happened if I had not ended up in the hospital.

Ruth

It is a really good idea to have a friend who understands you are bipolar and will help you out if you get into trouble. After an extremely bad episode, I was involuntarily admitted into a psychiatric hospital. After three days of being on medication and "coming to my senses," I called my friend Joe and told him where I was and that I needed to get out of there and back to work. Joe drove to the hospital and talked to my doctor and vouched for me, told the doctor I was a sales manager and had a good job. They discharged me and I will be forever grateful to Joe because he had my back and helped me out in my time of need.

Jane

There's very little reason to go to a psychiatric hospital other than being suicidal or psychotic and wanting not to end up dead or injured. You do not receive therapy that's better than what you can get outside, and you'll almost certainly be heavily medicated. In fact, in many places you do not get individual therapy at all. If you want help, you should find a normal therapist. It's a very incorrect idea that institutionalization is more intensive and will help you more. In fact, it will probably help you less. Being in your own home, in your own environment that you can control, facing the real problems of everyday life, you will be much more comfortable than staying in a place where you have no privacy, where nurses and staff treat you in a very condescending manner.

Scott

The benefits of being in the hospital for me include [these]: You are in a controlled environment in the event of physical violence or attempted suicide. It gives you a chance to regroup and get stabilized. It removes you from stress of relationships—spouse, significant other, kids. It is a forgivable excuse for missing work and may keep you from getting fired.

When you are sensible enough, call your boss and tell him what has happened. Typically companies have guidelines for health-related situations and your boss will likely involve human resources. The staff and doctors generally treat you well and take your craziness in stride. The food is usually decent. Finally, it's amazing how fast you can regain balance by taking medication.

Reasons to Check into a Psychiatric Hospital

- You have thoughts of hurting yourself or others.
- You are having hallucinations.
- You feel unsafe, like you are going to lose control and start beating your head against the wall or attack someone.
- You have bizarre or paranoid ideas (delusions).
- You have not eaten or slept for several days.
- You have serious problems with alcohol or drugs.
- You are thinking or talking too fast, jumping from topic to topic, or not making sense.
- You feel too exhausted or too depressed to get out of bed or take care of yourself or your family.
- You have tried outpatient treatment (therapy, medication, and support) and still have symptoms that interfere with your life.
- You need to make a major change in your treatment or medication under the close supervision of your doctor.

Voluntary Check-in

Approximately 75 percent of admissions into psychiatric hospitals are voluntary. Here are three ways to check into a psychiatric hospital:

1) Go directly to the psychiatric hospital and tell them you need to be admitted. They will then ask you questions, and based on your answers and the amount of available space, they will admit you or deny you. Most times, if you say you are suicidal at your evaluation, that's sufficient for immediate admittance.

2) Go to the emergency room of a hospital and tell them exactly what's going on. They will transport you to a psychiatric hospital.

3) Work with your psychiatrist to be admitted.

When you arrive at the psychiatric hospital, you will go to the Screening and Admissions Unit, where you will be asked to sign a voluntary evaluation and admission form. Next, you will be examined by a hospital physician; if the physician agrees that you should be hospitalized, you will be admitted.

Involuntary Commitment

Involuntary commitment (aka civil commitment or involuntary civil commitment) is the act of placing individuals in a psychiatric hospital or similar facility without their consent. Although such action may seem harsh, it is sometimes necessary in order to prevent people from harming themselves or others and to ensure that appropriate treatment is administered to them.

Hopefully by following the battle plan outlined in this book, you can successfully battle bipolar disorder and will never end up in this situation. Involuntary commitment is discussed in detail in chapter 11, "Legal Rights."

How Hospitalization Can Help

- The hospital is a safe place where you can begin to get well. It is a place to get away from the stresses that may be worsening your mood disorder and symptoms.
- It's a private way to get help when you need it. You don't have to tell anyone from outside the hospital where you are, even your family, if you choose not to.
- You can work with professionals to stabilize your severe symptoms, keep yourself safe, and learn new ways to cope with your illness.
- You can talk about traumatic experiences and explore your thoughts, ideas, and feelings openly.
- You can learn more about events, people, or situations that may trigger your manic or depressive episodes and how to cope with or avoid them.
- You may find a new treatment or combination of treatments that work.
- You will have time to reflect on your current battle plan and what improvements you can make.

What You Need to Know about Psychiatric Hospitals

- It is up to the psychiatrist(s) treating you to decide whether you can be discharged from the hospital. They grant you permission to leave. You can't just check out.
- You can make a reasonable number of phone calls.
- You have the legal right to decide who can visit you and must sign a form giving them the right to do so.
- Your medicine will be dispensed to you at set times, and a staff member will verify that you take the medicine.
- You will have to follow a schedule. There will be set times for meals, treatments, medications, activities, and bedtime.
- You may have physical or mental health tests. You may have blood tests to determine your medication levels or look for other physical problems that may be worsening your illness.
- You might have to ask for things you need more than once.
- Make sure that the doctor and the staff know about any other illnesses you have or medications you take. Be sure that you receive these medications.
- Your prescribing doctor may not be able to see you right away. You will probably talk to several different doctors, nurses, and staff members while you're on the ward.
- You will meet other people who are working to overcome their own problems and interact with them. Treat them with courtesy and respect, regardless of

what they may say or do. If someone is making you feel uncomfortable or unsafe, tell a staff member.
- Some of the people you meet may be able to relate to you and what you are going through. It may be a way for you to build or strengthen your support group.
- You may be in a locked ward. At first you may not be able to leave the ward. Later, you may be able to go to other parts of the hospital or get a pass to leave the hospital for a short time.
- You may have jewelry, personal care items, belts, shoelaces, or other personal belongings locked away during your stay. You may not be allowed to have items with glass or sharp edges, such as picture frames, CD cases, or spiral notebooks.
- You may share a room with someone else.
- In many places, the staff will not allow you to stay in your room for extended periods of time during the day. If you stay in your room, they may assume you are isolating yourself and keep you hospitalized until you can force yourself to stay with the other patients for a major portion of the day for several days.
- Hospital staff may check on you or interview you periodically.
- After you begin to recover and heal, you can request to transition from the hospital to an outpatient facility, which you attend during the day and are on your own for the rest of the time.

CHAPTER 11
Legal Rights

Note: The information presented in this chapter is an overview of legal rights based on material found on the Internet. Legal rights for the mentally ill vary by state and by country. Always consult a lawyer who is versed in the laws where you live for legal help. (Some lawyers will give a free consultation.)

The Laws Governing Involuntary Commitment

Involuntary commitment is a legal process through which an individual with symptoms of severe mental illness is court-ordered into treatment in a psychiatric hospital against his or her will. In general, laws restrict involuntary commitment to those who are "mentally ill" and/or under the influence of drugs or alcohol and are deemed to be in imminent danger of harming themselves or others.

If the police are called to a location, for whatever reason, and observe that you are suicidal, belligerent, threatening, or physically violent, they may take you to a psychiatric hospital or they may take you to jail. The immediate safety of you and anyone else is the primary concern. If you are bipolar, you should be taken to a mental health facility for evaluation instead of a jail cell. However, many times the police won't realize you are mentally ill. If you end up in jail due to a bipolar episode, tell the police and your lawyer that you are bipolar. You do have rights!

Whether you are taken to a mental health facility or jail, it's important to realize that you are not making a rational decision to act inappropriately. Your brain has betrayed you with bipolar disorder and you have become out of control, causing you to need law enforcement to keep yourself and those around you safe.

Here are three reasons you could be involuntarily committed to a psychiatric hospital.

1. You attempt suicide or become violent toward yourself.

When people are depressed, they're more likely to become violent toward themselves and attempt suicide. You can be involuntarily committed to a mental health facility if you attempt suicide or physically harm yourself.

2. You are aggressive and violent toward others.

Many of us who are bipolar have a history of explosive behavior. Some may call this rage, mania, violence, or anger. When people are manic, they are more likely to become aggressive and violent with others. The outburst itself is generally not premeditated; it is often triggered by some incident that is a climax of the build-up of fear, shame, guilt, or whatever strong emotions they are battling at the time.

3. A family member or someone you know has you committed.

With most adverse bipolar behavior, those most affected are usually the people who are closest to the bipolar individual, like family or friends. If you are having a bipolar episode and are violent, suicidal, or making threats, a family member or friend may decide to take action and have you committed to a psychiatric hospital.

At the time, it will most likely seem harsh. These types of cases of involuntary committal are usually accompanied by strong emotions of the person committed and the person responsible for the committing. It is highly possible that this person is taking this action because he or she loves you and wants to keep you, and perhaps themselves or others, safe until the episode runs its course.

If someone is attempting to have you committed to a psychiatric hospital against your will, get a lawyer. Bipolar episodes are scary, confusing, and heart wrenching. It is definitely to your advantage to consult with someone who is not emotionally involved to steer you through the legal issues and protect your legal rights.

In the rare case that the person who is attempting to have you involuntarily committed is trying to do you harm instead of help you, keep your wits about you as much as possible and, again, get a lawyer. Maybe you have not been getting along with that person and he or she is on the warpath against you. Do your best to remain calm and collected when you come before the judge and convince him or her that there is no reason to put you in the hospital and explain why the person is making things up. Your psychiatrist will be your best advocate in court.

Someone who decides to have you involuntarily committed to a psychiatric hospital must take the following steps:

- File an affidavit with the clerk of superior court or magistrate of district court. The clerk or magistrate may issue an order to a law enforcement officer to take you into custody for examination by a qualified professional.
- If the qualified professional finds that you are "mentally ill," you will be taken to a psychiatric hospital.
- When you arrive at the hospital you will be examined by a psychiatrist; if the hospital psychiatrist agrees with the first examiner that hospitalization is necessary, you will be admitted for observation and treatment. If he or she does not believe you should be in the hospital, you will be released.
- A court hearing must be held no later than ten days after you are taken into custody. The hearing may be held either in the county where the commitment was started or at the hospital. Within a few days after you are admitted, a lawyer from the Office of Special Counsel will contact you. He or she will be your lawyer at the initial hearing. You may also hire a lawyer at your own expense. At the hearing, the judge will decide whether you should be treated in the hospital or discharged. If you are committed, the judge will decide how many days you will be kept in the hospital before another hearing must be held.

At the hearing, you have the following rights:

- the right to an attorney (you may hire your own, or an attorney can be provided for you)
- the right to be present at the hearing
- the right to speak for yourself
- the right to challenge what is said about you

Legal Rights When in the Psychiatric Hospital

If you find yourself in a psychiatric hospital, you have the following rights:

- It is your legal right that the hospital staff verbally explains and provides you a written copy of the privacy policy, which gives you the right to choose whether you want to have visitors or not. If there are certain people you do not wish to see or hear from, the staff will ask you to write down their names, and they will make a note of it. If you do not wish to have outside friends, family members, employers, or anyone else know you're there, the staff will not make your presence known. They will not verify in any way that you are a patient there.
- You may immediately make telephone calls in order to get help with legal, medical, and mental health issues.
- You have the right to be visited by your clergy, lawyer, or physician at any time.
- You have the right to ask for help from hospital staff to make sure your rights are honored.
- You have the right to a civil commitment hearing, where a judge will decide whether you should be hospitalized by court order. You have the right to

a court-appointed attorney at the court hearing. It is highly recommended to have a lawyer represent you at a court hearing to protect your legal rights.
- You have the right to hire your own lawyer.
- You have the right to an independent expert evaluation of your mental condition. If you can't afford this evaluation, it must be provided to you at no charge.
- You have the right to file a grievance with the hospital if you feel your rights have been violated. You can request the hospital's clients' rights officer for help in filing your grievance.
- There is no time limit on a voluntary inpatient stay, and you may stay as long as you are willing and the medical staff believes there is a continued need for inpatient treatment.
- You may communicate by sealed mail with any individual, group, or agency.
- You have the right to be furnished with writing materials and reasonable postage.
- You have the right to receive mail, unless the head of the hospital determines it is medically harmful for you to receive mail; all such correspondence will be returned unopened to sender with an explanation signed by the head of the hospital.
- You have the right to receive visitors at regular hours, unless the head of the hospital determines it is medically harmful for you to receive visitors and so informs family and other visitors. They must also be notified immediately when you have recovered sufficiently to receive visitors.
- You have the right to wear your own clothes.
- You have the right to keep and use personal possessions, including toilet articles.

- You have the right to request to be released from the hospital.

Can I Be Forced to Take Medication?

The standard procedure for dealing with medication refusal is to take the patient to court to legally force him to agree to take it. At the trial, the psychiatrist will explain exactly why he or she thinks the patient needs to be hospitalized and why it is important for the patient to take medicine. The judge then rules that the patient either has to take medication or doesn't have to take it. If so, this means that, even if the patient refuses his medication, he is legally obligated to take it. When he returns to the psych hospital, the doctors will offer him oral meds first, but if he will not take them, staff members will physically restrain him and administer the medicine.

How Do I Get Discharged from the Hospital?

If you check yourself into a psychiatric hospital voluntarily and you decide you want to be discharged, you cannot simply sign yourself out and leave when you decide to do so. There is a process that must be followed. You can request to be discharged by filling out the right paperwork. If the request for discharge is approved, you will be allowed to leave within three workdays (Monday through Friday, not weekends or holidays). If you request to be discharged, there are three possible outcomes:

- The psychiatrist who is handling your case will agree that you can leave. When your request to be

discharged is granted, you can leave at the end of seventy-two hours.
- There are cases in which someone who admitted himself voluntarily to the psych hospital is not allowed to leave of his own accord because the doctors and staff feel he is harmful to himself or others. In this case, the hospital staff can ask the court to commit you. The hospital staff must file papers (an affidavit) within three workdays of receiving your "request of discharge" form. Your request for release becomes a request for a hearing. You will receive notice of a court hearing before a judge to determine whether a court order will be issued to keep you in the hospital. At the hearing, if the judge rules that you need to stay in the hospital, you become an involuntary patient; otherwise, you will be discharged.
- If the hospital does not file an affidavit within three workdays, you must be released immediately.

The Benefits of Having a Psychiatric Advance Directive

In order to protect yourself from a devastating outcome of future bipolar episodes, you can prepare a Psychiatric Advance Directive (PAD). The PAD is a legal contract that allows you to choose and control in advance the care you will receive when you are mentally incapacitated and unable to direct your own care during times of crisis.

The PAD serves to inform others about what treatment you want or don't want from psychiatrists or other mental health professionals in the event of a bipolar episode, and it can identify a person to whom you have given authority to make

Bipolar Battle Plan

decisions on your behalf. Instead of having some stranger make the decisions or have your family guess at what you would want, you can list your preferences.

Typical provisions in a PAD include the following:

- a list of symptoms you might experience during a period of crisis
- if you have kids, the person or people you want to take care of them
- medication instructions, including a list of medications to be given ("I agree to these meds," "I don't agree to these meds")
- other info about medications, allergies, side effects
- your choice of hospital
- list of emergency contacts (doctors, family member, or friend)
- crisis precipitants: "The following may cause me to have a bipolar episode."
- protective factors: "The following may help me avoid a mental health crisis."
- preferences for ways the staff can help you while you are there
- list of people who can visit you in the hospital
- what you want to be taken care of at your home if you are hospitalized (pets, plants, children, etc.)
- preference as to whether special therapies can be used—for example electroconvulsive therapy (ECT)

Almost all states permit some form of legal advance directive for health care, which can be used to direct psychiatric treatment. Consult a lawyer in your state to help prepare a PAD that specifies your personal wishes and requirements.

The Americans with Disabilities Act

The Americans with Disabilities Act (ADA) is a law that gives civil rights protection to individuals with disabilities. The ADA's legal definition of a disability is especially beneficial to those with bipolar disorder. According to the US Equal Employment Opportunity Commission, the ADA defines the term *disability* as "a physical or mental impairment that substantially limits a major life activity." Since bipolar disorder seriously affects people's ability to work, the ADA is of vital importance to those with the disorder. It ensures that people with bipolar disorder have rights at work and, in serious cases, provides them with disability benefits if they are unable to work due to their condition. Note that there are some restrictions that may apply in specific circumstances. If your work is being affected by bipolar disorder, investigate the ADA.

CHAPTER 12
Winning the Bipolar War

Controlling the symptoms of bipolar disorder is an ongoing process. You must be relentless about getting necessary treatment and sticking to it. This book has detailed a bipolar battle plan that can help you learn to cope with your emotions, control negative thinking, minimize physical symptoms, deal with medication issues, manage problems of everyday life, and come to terms with having bipolar disorder.

Remember that the first rule of combat is that all battle plans get altered. Be prepared to make changes as time goes on. Change your plan as many times as needed until you achieve optimal mental and physical health.

Make the commitment to become a warrior, master the weapons in the bipolar battle plan, and win the war against bipolar disorder. Winning the war means never having another out-of-control bipolar episode that causes you to harm someone else, attempt suicide, mutilate yourself, wreck your finances, lose your job, destroy relationships with friends and loved ones, or destroy your health. Winning the war means living a productive, happy life and making your dreams come true!

Bipolar Battle Plan Summary

- Create a contingency plan and use it.
- Monitor your mood (emotions and feelings).
- Be vigilant for bipolar symptoms.
- Optimize your medications.
- Hire a good psychiatrist whom you trust.
- Bipolar, heal thyself (take responsibility for your own treatment).
- Never stop learning about bipolar disorder.
- Exercise, eat healthily, and take vitamins.
- Don't abuse alcohol and drugs (or do go from too much to not too much).
- Use your team (psychiatrist, support groups, friends, and family).
- Strengthen and train your mind.
- Be aware of your legal rights.
- Be knowledgeable of psychiatric hospitals.
- Don't settle—do what it takes to make your dreams come true.

You have all the weapons you need—now fight!

HELPFUL RESOURCES

Ten Best iPhone and Android Apps for Bipolar Disorder
- http://www.healthline.com/health-slideshow/top-iphone-android-apps-bipolar-disorder#1

National Institute of Mental Health (NIMH): The mission of the NIMH is to transform the understanding and treatment of mental illnesses through basic and clinical research, paving the way for prevention, recovery, and cure.
- http://www.nimh.nih.gov/index.shtml

Black Dog Institute: An educational, research, and clinical facility offering specialized expertise in mood disorders.
- http://www.blackdoginstitute.org.au/healthprofessionals/gps/
- onlinetrainingprogram.cfm

BP Magazine: An excellent quarterly magazine about bipolar disorder that also comes in an online version and has a great online forum, making it easy to ask questions and get answers.
- http://www.bphope.com/

Wikipedia is a free online encyclopedia with an excellent overview and description of bipolar disorder.
- http://en.wikipedia.org/wiki/Bipolar_disorder

PsychEducation: Extensive mental health information on specific topics.
- http://www.psycheducation.org/

NeuroStar TMS: Transcranial magnetic stimulation therapy is an FDA-cleared non-invasive medical treatment that is specifically for patients with major depression who have not benefited from initial antidepressant medication.
- http://neurostar.com/nondrug-treatment-for-depression/?gclid=CNa_na6hi7QCFQf0nAodBigAoA
- http://www.youtube.com/NeurostarTMSTherapy

Dbsalliance.org: Depression and Bipolar Support Alliance
- http://www.dbsalliance.org/site/PageServer?pagename=home

"Non-Medical Treatment for Bipolar Disorder." Article in ehow.com.
- http://www.ehow.com/facts_5685287_non_medical-treatment-bipolar-disorder.html#ixzz1xPMeZGdE

"What Part of the Brain Does Bipolar II Disorder Affect?" Article in ehow.com showing which areas of the brain are affected by bipolar disorder and their specific impact:
- http://www.ehow.com/about_5642046_part-bipolar-ii-disorder-affect.html#ixzz29t7raPdR

Newharbinger Publications: Excellent source on Mood Disorders.
- http://www.newharbinger.com

Physicians Desktop Reference
- http://www.pdrhealth.com

BIBLIOGRAPHY

"Carlos Castaneda's Don Juan Teachings." Accessed June 6, 2013. http://www.prismagems.com/castaneda/donjuan8.html.

Caruso, Kevin. 2009. "Bipolar Disorder and Suicide." Suicide.org. Accessed June 6, 2013. http://www.suicide.org/bipolar-disorder-and-suicide.html.

Castaneda, Carlos. 1998. *The Wheel of Time.* New York: Pocket Books.

Cowen, Mark. 2011. "Life Expectancy Reduced in Schizophrenia, Bipolar Disorder Patients." Accessed June 6, 2013.
http://www.medwirenews.com/47/93550/Psychiatry/Life_expectancy_reduced_in_schizophrenia,_bipolar_disorder_patients.html.

Evans, Dwight. 2000. "Bipolar Disorder." Accessed June 1, 2013.
http://www.brainexplorer.org/bipolar_disorder/Bipolar_Disorder_%20comorbidity.shtml.

Feather, Ken. 1995. *On the Toltec Path.* VT: Bear & Company.

Ghaemi, Nassir. 2011. "Positive Aspects of Mental Illness: A Review on Bipolar Disorder." Accessed March 5, 2013. http://www.bphope.com/item.aspx/915/accentuate-the-positive.

Haycock, Dean. 2010. *The Everything Health Guide to Adult Bipolar Disorder.* MA: Adams Media.

Hill, Napoleon. 1997. *Napoleon Hill's Keys to Success.* New York: Plume.

Hornbacher, Marya. 2008. *Madness: A Bipolar Life.* New York: First Mariner Books.

Jamison, Kay. 1996. *An Unquiet Mind.* New York: First Vintage Books.

—. 1994. *Touched with Fire.* New York: Free Press Paperbacks.

Kessler, R. C. 2005. "The Numbers Count: Mental Disorders in America." Accessed March 10, 2013. http://www.nimh.nih.gov/health/publications/the-numbers-count-mental-disorders-in-america/index.shtml.

Mariant, David. "Surviving Bipolar." Accessed February 14, 2013. http://www.survivingbipolar.com/green_suicide.htm#2.

Martin, B. 2006. "Phases and Symptoms of Bipolar Disorder." *Psych Central.* Accessed January 14, 2012. http://psychcentral.com/lib/2006/phases-and-symptoms-of-bipolar-disorder/.

McElroy, S. L. 2002. "Correlates of Overweight and Obesity in 644 Patients with Bipolar Disorder." Accessed September 2, 2012.
http://www.ncbi.nlm.nih.gov/pubmed/11926719.

Monson, Kristi. 2007a. "Risperdal Side Effects." Accessed April 10, 2013.
http://schizophrenia.emedtv.com/risperdal/risperdal-side-effects.html.

—. 2007b. "Wellbutrin Side Effects." Accessed November 12, 2012.
http://depression.emedtv.com/wellbutrin/wellbutrin-side-effects.html.

Narita, Kosuke. 2011. "Volume Reduction of Ventromedial Prefrontal Cortex in Bipolar II Patients with Rapid Cycling: A Voxel-Based Morphometric Study." Accessed July 7, 2013.
http://www.sciencedirect.com/science/article/pii/S0278584610004616

Novick, Swartz, and H. A. Frank. 2010. "Suicide Attempts in Bipolar I and Bipolar II Disorder: A Review and Meta-analysis of the Evidence." Accessed April 13, 2013.
http://onlinelibrary.wiley.com/doi/10.1111/j.1399-5618.2009.00786.x/abstract;jsessionid=21AE4997510C8267D6B03A995F9F54F9.d04t01.

Purse, Marcia. 2009. "Anxiety Medications: Bipolar Disorder Medications Library." Accessed January 16, 2013.
http://bipolar.about.com/od/sedatives/a/anxiety_medications.htm.

Ruiz, Miguel. 1997. "The Four Agreements." San Rafael: Amber-Allen Publishing. Accessed March 14, 2013. http://www.bodhitree.com/lectures/Don.Miguel.Ruiz.html.

Sachs, Gary. 2008. "Are Men or Women More Likely to Develop Bipolar Disorder?" Accessed June 6, 2013. http://abcnews.go.com/Health/BipolarRiskFactors/story?id=4356077.

Thompson, Dennis. 2010. "Can Bipolar Lead to Diabetes?" Accessed November 12, 2012.
http://www.everydayhealth.com/bipolar-disorder/can-bipolar-disorder-lead-to-diabetes.aspx.

University of Michigan General Research Center. 2005. "Evidence of Brain Chemistry Abnormalities in Bipolar Disorder." Accessed March 4, 2013.
http://bipolar.about.com/cs/menu_science/a/press_umich0210.htm.

Vann, Madeline. 2010. "Are People with Bipolar Disorder Dangerous?" Accessed March 5, 2013.
http://www.everydayhealth.com/bipolar-disorder/are-people-with-bipolar-disorder-dangerous.aspx.

APPENDIX

The individuals below who are currently living (Kay Jamison, Catherine Zeta-Jones, Jean-Claude Van Damme) have publicly announced that they are bipolar. The individuals who are no longer living are speculated to have been bipolar based on symptoms they exhibited.

Marilyn Monroe
Chapter 1, Lead Photo:
http://commons.wikimedia.org/wiki/File:Marilyn_Monroe,_The_Prince_and_the_Showgirl,_1.jpg
Chapter 1, Lead Quote:
http://www.brainyquote.com/quotes/authors/m/marilyn_monroe.html

Abraham Lincoln
Chapter 3, Lead Photo:
http://commons.wikimedia.org/wiki/File:Abraham_Lincoln_seated,_Feb_9,_1864.jpg
Chapter 3, Lead Quote:
http://www.brainyquote.com/quotes/authors/a/abraham_lincoln.html

Catherine Zeta-Jones
Chapter 4, Lead Photo:
http://commons.wikimedia.org/wiki/File:Catherine_Zeta-Jones_Feb05.jpg
Chapter 4, Lead Quote:
http://www.huffingtonpost.com/2013/05/21/catherine-zeta-jones-bipolar-treatment_n_3312701.html
Documented sources that Zeta-Jones is bipolar:
http://www.forbes.com/sites/markpasetsky/2011/04/20/catherine-zeta-jones-bipolar-battle-is-peoples-cover-why-readers-will-buy-it/

Kay Jamison
Chapter 5, Lead Photo:
http://commons.wikimedia.org/wiki/File:JAMISON754.JPG
Chapter 5, Lead Quote:
http://www.goodreads.com/author/quotes/19038.Kay_Redfield_Jamison
Documented source that Jamison is bipolar:
http://en.wikipedia.org/wiki/Kay_Jamison

Winston Churchill
Chapter 6, Lead Photo:
http://commons.wikimedia.org/wiki/File:Winston_Churchill_cph.3b13157.jpg
Chapter 6, Lead Quote:
http://www.brainyquote.com/quotes/authors/w/winston_churchill.html

Jean-Claude Van Damme
Chapter 7, Lead Photo:
http://commons.wikimedia.org/wiki/File:Jean-Claude_Van_Damme_June_2,_2007.jpg
Chapter 7, Lead Quote:

http://www.brainyquote.com/quotes/authors/j/jean_claude_van_damme.html
Documented source that Van Damme is bipolar:
http://bipolar.about.com/cs/celebs/a/jeanclaude.htm
Jean Claude Van Damme says he is bipolar (manic depressive):
http://bipolar-disorder.mywisdombase.com/Articles/Famous_People_with_Bipolar_Disorder_Is_Adversity_the_Source_of_Creativity.php

Isaac Newton
Chapter 8, Lead Photo:
http://commons.wikimedia.org/wiki/File:Sir_Isaac_Newton_by_Sir_Godfrey_Kneller,_Bt.jpg
Chapter 8, Lead Quote:
http://www.brainyquote.com/quotes/authors/i/isaac_newton.html

Theodore Roosevelt
Chapter 9, Lead Photo:
http://commons.wikimedia.org/wiki/File:Theodore_Roosevelt-Harris_and_Ewing.jpg
Chapter 9, Lead Quote:
http://www.brainyquote.com/quotes/authors/t/theodore_roosevelt.html

MY PERSONAL CONTINGENCY PLAN

Name:
Phone:
Address:

Support People　　　　　　**Name**　　　　**Phone Number**

Support Person 1 (Psychiatrist)

Support Person 2

Support Person 3

24-Hour Emergency Numbers

1)

2)

3)

Current Medications

1)

2)

3)

Medication Contingency Plan

1)

2)

3)

Things That May Trigger a Relapse

1)

2)

3)

4)

Mania Early Warning Signs

1)

2)

3)

4)

Depression Early Warning Signs

1)

2)

3)

4)

If I develop any of these signs, I will . . .

1)

2)

3)

4)

If my support people observe these signs, they may . . .

1)

2)

3)

4)

I have a psychiatric advanced directive.

YES   NO

If "yes," attach it or note where it is; if "no," one should be created in case of emergency.

Signed:

Date:

Witness:

Remember to make a few copies of this for your most trusted friends and family to have and use, just in case.

A plan is useless if not put in place!

PERSONAL NOTES

PERSONAL NOTES

PERSONAL NOTES

PERSONAL NOTES